skin
sense

Beauty is a Vibe

Love
Dr. Kiran

Praise for Dr Kiran Sethi

Dr Kiran is a world-class skincare guru. I love how she integrates nutrition and wellness into her recommendations. Her approach is truly beauty from inside and out, and that's a game changer. I love this book about her work!

– **Dr Amy Shah**, double board-certified MD and nutritionist

Dr Kiran Lohia is a magician! She knows her craft inside-out and is easily one of the best skin doctors I have ever been to. Always good to know that she's there to help maintain my glow.

–**Riya Sen**, actress

Dr Kiran explains beauty and aesthetics in an integrative and easy-to-approach way that embodies the true sense of beauty from the inside-out … This book is a winner!

– **Dr Vishakha Shivdasani**, physician and award-winning nutritionist

Dr Kiran Lohia is an accomplished name to reckon with in the aesthetic industry. Her natural flair for delivering cutting-edge technology and innovative treatment plans makes her much sought after. It's been a pleasure to associate with her over the years on numerous platforms and I wish her every success.

– **Dr Malavika Kohli**, dermatologist

skin sense

DR KIRAN'S GUIDE TO BEING BEAUTFUL

dr kiran sethi

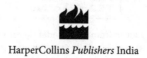

HarperCollins *Publishers* India

First published in India by HarperCollins *Publishers* 2022
4th Floor, Tower A, Building No. 10, Phase II, DLF Cyber City,
Gurugram, Haryana – 122002
www.harpercollins.co.in

2 4 6 8 10 9 7 5 3 1

Copyright © Dr Kiran Sethi 2022

P-ISBN: 978-93-5489-375-9
E-ISBN: 978-93-5489-383-4

The views and opinions expressed in this book are the author's own
and the facts are as reported by her, and the publishers
are not in any way liable for the same.

Kiran Sethi asserts the moral right
to be identified as the author of this work.

All rights reserved. No part of this publication may be reproduced,
stored in a retrieval system, or transmitted, in any form or by any
means, electronic, mechanical, photocopying, recording or otherwise,
without the prior permission of the publishers.

Typeset in 11.5/15.2 Arno Pro at
Manipal Technologies Limited, Manipal

Printed and bound at
Thomson Press (India) Ltd

🅕🅘◎🅞 HarperCollinsIn

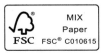

This book is produced from independently certified FSC® paper
to ensure responsible forest management.

This book is dedicated to my daughter, my light, my boss
Raina
And my family

CONTENTS

1

INTRODUCTION

MIRROR, MIRROR, ON THE WALL

Beauty begins the moment you decide to be yourself.

– Coco Chanel

I still remember an Indian aunty telling me she was glad I had lost weight because she feared I would never get married. I was fourteen. Many women are subjected to the same scrutiny and no-holds-barred criticism that makes them feel like they will never match up to the flawless images on social media and television. But you are not alone. Billions of people around the world are made to feel the same way. Is it fair? Absolutely not!

Feeling beautiful isn't easy. I have met maybe two people in my life who have told me that they feel beautiful. Celebrities, socialites, Instagram stars, models alike suffer the same insecurities that all of us do, if not more. And everyone famous spends way more time on their appearance than you do, I can assure you. That is a function of their job. They have to look perfect at nearly all times. They have to make sure they don't have any flaws that show up from a variety of camera angles. I can also tell you that they do not 'wake up like that'. I know, their social media profiles make them look über confident, like they own the world. Hate to break it to you, but it isn't true. In fact, the level of their insecurity regarding appearance, no matter how beautiful they are, can rival that of your teenage sister or daughter. And the fact that they have millions of Instagram followers who would kill to look like them probably doesn't bring them much solace from the insecurity either. When your perception of beauty becomes one that derives from those of these influencers and celebrities, social media, television shows, movies, magazines, bloggers, the beauty and fashion industry – all earn money off this concept. If you are made to feel insecure, perhaps you will buy into the latest trend. 'Hey, this month it's the Kardashian cheekbone, while next month, it'll be the sculpted eyebrow' – there is never any rest from the continuous barrage of beauty must-haves. The pressure just does not let up. So, while perhaps you were fine with that little hook on your nose before, the latest Bollywood nose job tells you, 'Hey, maybe there is something wrong with the way you look.' And you think, maybe I need to change in order to fit into this beauty ideal so that people will feel I am worthy. Now it's not only our surrounding media but also the peer pressure. In India (and in the rest of Asia too, by the way), casually commenting on a person's appearance is so common that people often don't realize it can be rude and hurtful.

Now, while you may be feeling insecure thinking, 'Hey, that guy won't like me unless I have this desirable pout,' that guy may be concerned with the size of his biceps and wouldn't even be paying attention to the imagined flaws in your lips. Each and every person has insecurities that are ever-burgeoning, but there will never be any permanent solution to them because there will always be something new to worry about. The point is that while you are thinking you look terrible and everyone is staring at that zit on your nose, the likelihood is that they are more concerned with the size of their own noses or their pores or perhaps that mole at the corner of their lip. So, maybe the first step to beauty is not zapping that zit or correcting that supposed imperfection; maybe it is self-awareness, perspective and self-worth.

Since I am an MD from the US, and a physician specializing in skin and aesthetics, you must be thinking, 'This chick is crazy! Why shouldn't we fix what is making us feel insecure?' That's not what I am saying. I am saying you should first take a step back and recognize that people with zits, pores, stretch marks, wrinkles, sagging skin, weight gain issues and more are all normal and have the ability to be happy within their skin. We as humans don't need external validation. We need to learn to cultivate internal validation. We need to understand that getting rid of our pigmentation will not intrinsically change how we feel about ourselves. I have clients who have come to me with their families, fiancées, friends and said, 'I do not leave the house or go out with my friends because I feel so ashamed of my skin.' That concept upsets me deeply. Skin problems are problems that can be solved! That is what I am here for! Just like any other problem, they don't mean anything beyond that. And I am here to tell you that you are worthy no matter what you look like. That is a fact and has been proven throughout history. So, let's not allow our insecurities to take away from our everyday living. Let's spend some time appreciating what we have and feeling strong. And, simultaneously, we can zap zits.

While we must all remind ourselves of our self-worth, which has nothing to do with appearance, it doesn't mean we still can't act on our aesthetic concerns. Pimples, when not treated early enough, can cause severe scars. Stretch marks can be a reminder of a painful miscarriage. We have the right to do what we can to deal with things that bother us or serve as a reminder of a painful experience. I have had two miscarriages myself, one was when I was seven months pregnant. My body has never felt the same since, and I struggle with that. Women with scars or discolouration still feel the hurt when their appearance is commented upon. It is one thing to accept ourselves, but another to say 'I have to live with it' when there is a multitude of solutions out there.

So, let's get down and dirty now. Okay, I don't mean sex (although, not going to lie, good sex totally helps with making you feel gorgeous!). What I mean is, let's get down to the brass tacks. How do we work on feeling internally validated while also getting our glow on? In this book, I am going to talk to you about how to get LIT from within.

First things first, a little about myself and why you should even bother reading this book. So, I was born and brought up in New York. I was raised in Long Island by a mom who is a Type-A mom and a doctor and a powerhouse businessman dad. I went to Columbia University, followed by med school, and then did my medical training at Mount Sinai Beth Israel in downtown Manhattan. After that, I went on to earn a graduate degree in dermatology, American board certifications in aesthetics & lasers, and a diplomate in cosmetic formulation on the by and by. I have treated celebrities from Hollywood and Bollywood. I have also cared for thousands of poor, underserved patients from Kolkata and Eastern India through my work with slums and free clinics, and have seen the most terrible mutilating skin diseases that you could imagine. But I have also seen hope, strength, self-worth and confidence even through the worst.

I have been in India for about ten years now, and have experienced the entire gamut of clients and client experiences. When I moved to India, I was a firm believer in allopathy and medication as the only line of treatment. I thought this is what I know and this is the only way to be. Whoa, was I wrong! Living in India, I was exposed to an entirely different and holistic way of thinking when the first questions I was always asked were, 'Doc, what am I eating wrong? How can I change my diet to improve my skin?' Trust me, that is not what patients ask you in America. There, the questions tend to be more like: 'Will I look like Kim Kardashian after this?' And, 'Can I get some pain pills with that?' (I'm kidding … I promise it's not that bad). But those questions got me thinking – what was it that was so important in our lifestyle that could help explain these issues and help those looking to feel better about themselves? If you are willing to change your habits, then perhaps the world truly becomes your oyster.

Dietary alterations can help with a variety of conditions, from PCOS to acne to pigmentation to psoriasis to eczema to heart disease to even infertility! Thousands of studies have been published to the same effect. Furthermore, multivitamins have been proven to be essentially useless. It is food that can truly help heal and nourish us. In addition to this research, I have explored Ayurveda, homoeopathy, functional medicine, Chinese medicine, nutrition, psychology, biofeedback, and a variety of diets and dietary restrictions in my quest to discover how we can all be beautiful from the inside out. I have watched and listened to tens of thousands of patient stories, and researched each and every alternative therapy that they have been through that has given them success or failure. Further, I met and collaborated with a variety of functional medicine doctors, nutritionists, and naturopaths from around the world so that I could further hone my knowledge while tailoring it to the Indian population. I came out of it realizing that there is quite a bit of consensus amongst all of these disciplines when you really get down to it, and there is a damn lot more to learn.

So, basically, in addition to learning how to feel good about ourselves, we need to learn how to be good to ourselves. And that means changing how we live, eat, breathe and even move. First, we must accept ourselves for who we are and enjoy that state of existence. Eat to live, rather than living to eat unhealthily. Eating bad food is a habit; chips, sodas and desserts have been shown to create addictive chemical circuits in the brain. Food should not be a drug; it is designed to nourish us. Use it as it was intended. Already, the food and water we get are filled with toxic plastic derivatives, hormones, pesticides, insecticides, antibiotics, and more. What can we do to improve the situation that we are already stuck with? Luckily, there is so much, and I will tell you about them! It will also go beyond just food. Your body is designed to move and exercise. Use the muscles and physicality you were born with and move every day to increase blood flow and detoxification in the body. At the end of the day, we only have ourselves, and it is time to commit to that.

Now, in addition to all of this, we still may have to do more and take advantage of the science out there. Let's be honest, no amount of amla or adaptogenic mushrooms are going to erase those pores. You can eat flax seeds until Christmas, but all your acne and acne marks will not go away. So, who says everything has to be so hard? Trust me, there is no controversy. You can love natural eating and healthy living, and still take advantage of the latest aesthetic technology and laser off those lines and Botox those wrinkles – if that's what you wish. I can name a number of yoga teachers and meditation disciples who do just that. So, I am also going to chart out what you can do from the outside to help you realize just how hard you have been working on the inside! You will get the 411 on how to choose what skincare to buy, in addition to the treatments you can undergo. From peels, lasers, Botox, fillers, microneedling and more, you will learn what you can do at home and at your local cosmetologist or dermatologist's clinic. So do not fear, I am on top of making sure you can own that selfie with pride, while walking around with a major confident swagger. You will get to feel beautiful while looking beautiful. What could be better?

At the end of the day, I truly believe in each and every piece of advice in this book, and will teach my daughter the same as she grows up, hoping that the habits I instil in her will serve her throughout her life and will continue through further generations. I hope that she will crave broccoli instead of chocolate. (I have failed at that already, but I am still trying.) I pray she will want to exercise and be active throughout her life. I try to teach her mindfulness and engagement with every moment (even though I am addicted to Instagram myself). And finally, I hope that she will not feel ashamed of her body or her appearance. My dreams for my daughter will hopefully guide you in your quest to be LIT from within. Happy reading and get glowing already!

2

IN YOUR SKIN

EVERYTHING YOU NEED TO KNOW ABOUT YOUR SKIN

No heels, No shirt, No skirt,
All I'm in is just skin.
No jeans, take 'em off,
Wanna feel your skin.
You a beast, oh.
You know that I like that.
Come on baby,
All I wanna see you in is just skin.
All I wanna see you in is just skin.
All I wanna see you in is just skin.
Oooh
All I wanna see you in
All I wanna see you in is your skin, oh.
– 'Skin', Rihanna

The world stops at your skin! Quite literally. Your skin is the threshold that stops the outside world from merging with your inside. It is your outline, your sketch to the world. Everyone wants beautiful skin. In my entire career as an aesthetic and skin doctor, I have never met anyone who does not want beautiful skin. Am I right? Isn't that why you are reading this? Let's get you to it then!

What is beautiful skin? I know you all have heard of K-beauty, right? But Dr. K beauty is actually S-beauty, i.e., *Simple beauty*. I don't believe you need to apply twelve products to your skin every day. I believe in simplicity, and that's how I am going to approach this book. I want you all to understand your skin and hair, and approach your beauty with intelligence and a sense of curation. You are you, you are an individual, and you are fabulous. Don't let fear dictate your skincare. If you don't apply four separate essences in the morning, you will not end up with bad skin. I PROMISE! Trust me, simpler is better. Hence, S-BEAUTY baby!

As we go deeper into your skincare routines through this book, I will teach you how to do your skincare intuitively because, I believe intuitive skincare is actually simple skincare, which gives much better results. And, beautiful skin is skin that is healthy in every way. How do you get healthy skin? Well, for that, you will have to read the whole book! But let's start with getting to know your skin first.

WHAT IS SKIN?

The skin is the largest organ in your body. It protects you from the environment, while also balancing your internal body temperature. It is also an expression of whatever is happening inside your body. That is why skin is used to understand the overall health of your body. Problems such as iron deficiency, diabetes, inflammation, heart disease, and cancer can all show up on the skin and nails – reflecting the state of your health.

Skin is not just one layer though. There are three layers to skin – epidermis, dermis and hypodermis. The top-most layer that we can see is the epidermis. The line to remember here is: *the epidermis keeps you bright!* It consists of both living and dead skin cells and is as thin as a sheet of paper. As old skin cells die, newer ones push them to the epidermis layer. The quicker this process, the healthier your skin looks. Old skin cells from the deepest layer of the epidermis travel to the top-most layer and flake off to make way for new cells. The lifecycle of skin cells is about a month, and the body removes about 30,000-40,000 skin cells every day. Isn't it cool that you can literally shed your old skin? Our bodies are SO AMAZING!

This is the process of regeneration, which happens mainly in the epidermis layer. Another super important thing that the epidermis layer works on is: protecting your body. It keeps the bad stuff out and the good stuff in. The epidermis layer has these special immune system cells called Langerhans cells, which detect foreign substances and defend your body against infections, helping you stay healthy. That's not all; the epidermis layer also gives your skin its colour. It produces melanin, the thing that determines your skin colour and protects it against

UV rays. So, now you understand why you have to love and care for that epidermis layer of the skin?

The next layer is the dermis, which is the middle layer of the skin, below the epidermis and above the hypodermis. And it has all the elastin fibres and collagen that give your skin its strength and firmness. *The dermis keeps you tight, honey*! The dermis layer is also crucial because it makes you sweat. That's right, the sweat glands are located in the dermis layer of the skin. They produce sweat, which then travels through tiny openings called pores. Sweat may seem gross and greasy but it's actually your body's natural detox as it flushes out the toxins, alcohol and salt. It also keeps you cool. The dermis is also the layer in which you feel sensations. It has nerve endings, which send messages to the brain about how something feels: itchy, soft, painful, etc. It also produces hair and oil, besides bringing up blood to your skin that helps in regulating body temperature. Your dermis is a busy and important layer, and you must take care of it.

The bottom-most layer of the skin is the hypodermis, which contains fat, nerves and large blood vessels – keeping you strong and ready to fight! Its work is to provide oxygen and nutrition to the dermis layer and to also connect the skin to the bone and muscle beneath it. It is also our shock absorber and helps prevent injury. It is also the site of connective tissue and keeps you tight, too, so don't get confused.

That's the inside of our skin: three layers, all performing different tasks to keep you protected. Your skin has got you covered!

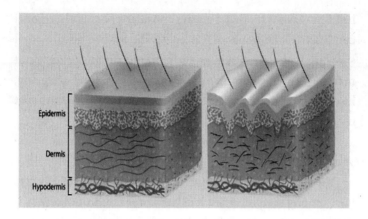

Here's a little poem for you all to remember your skin layers:

The epidermis keeps you bright
The dermis keeps you tight
Your hypodermis brings the fight.
Let's bring on some light!

I guess I am not a poet. But I do know skin!

However, although everyone's skin has the three layers, we do not all have identical skin. Like I said, you are you and your skin is as unique as you are. There are various skin types. How do you know what skin type you are? Let's find out!

Different types of skin

Basically, there are four different types of skin – normal, dry, oily, and combination. This is defined by the amount of sebum (oil) you make. If you are making too much sebum, there could be a few reasons for that. I always consider a possible hormonal condition. Conditions such as polycystic ovarian disease often show up with excess skin or scalp oiliness. If your skin is not making enough sebum and feels dry, then I look at ageing, history of eczema or any sensitivity issues, and incorrect product usage as causes.

So, let's understand how you can determine what skin type you have.

Those of you with combination skin types will typically also have an oily scalp or a tendency towards dandruff. Balancing your scalp sebum levels is the key to balancing your T-zone.

SKIN TYPE TISSUE TEST

First, cleanse your face with water or with a gentle cleanser that is non-foaming, like the Cetaphil cleanser or Episoft Cleanser.

Then wait an hour and see how your skin feels. Does it feel tight or stretchy? Does it wrinkle when you pinch it? If yes, it means your skin is dry.

Does it get shiny or greasy all over the face? When you pat it with a tissue or a blotting paper, do you see sebum on it? Does it feel smooth to touch? If yes, it is oily.

What if it is oily only on the T-zone but your cheeks are dry? (The T-zone is the area of the nose and forehead – forming a 'T' shape). If that is the case, then it is combination skin.

Finally, if your skin just feels fine – neither tight and stretchy nor shiny and greasy – and nothing comes off on the tissue or blotting paper, then you have normal skin. Ideally, the goal is to have normal skin: it means that your body is making just the right amount of sebum. But combination skin also falls within normal range so don't stress about that either!

Those are the skin types. Further, there are different adjectives you can add on to your skin type – such as sensitive, acne-prone, dehydrated – based on what you can see and feel. Let's discuss these adjectives you use to describe your skin when you talk to me.

Sensitive skin

What does it mean to have sensitive skin? Typically, this means you have rosacea, or a condition where your skin is ultra-reactive to different products or food and environmental triggers. It is closely associated with gut health. It can result in dry skin, although not always. It can also result in recurrent flushing or a sensation of heat in the skin, along with pimple-like lesions, enlarged pores and even skin flaking. It's important to know you can still have rosacea or sensitive skin with oily skin.

Acne-prone skin

What about acne-prone skin? Well, you can have a tendency to get acne no matter what skin type you have. Acne starts with recurrent blackheads or obstructed follicles, but often goes on to become whiteheads, bumps, little white-headed pustules, nodules and/or cysts. Different types of acne can exist at the same time and on any skin type. I have seen acne on both dry and oily skin.

Dehydrated skin

The last kind is dehydrated skin – this denotes how much water is retained in your skin, which is different from dry skin, where there is less sebum or oil production. Any skin type can have dehydrated skin, and it shows up as worsened fine lines, uneven skin texture or a lack of turgidity when you pull the skin. It happens from prolonged exposure to windy and cool or dry weather, air conditioners or heaters indoors, pollution, excess caffeine, and internal dehydration.

TYPES OF SKIN AND SKINCARE

So, how do you manage skincare for your specific skin type? Lucky for us, and contrary to popular belief, we don't really need to buy super-specialized products once our skin type is determined. Super-specialized products are a marketing myth designed to ensure people buy more products. My goal when I prescribe skincare is to actually help you balance your skin type, not continue to cause further imbalance. Let's run through what you really need as per your skin type.

Oily skin

A lot of people end up with excessively oily skin because of both internal and external factors. Internal factors may include stress, which results in the adrenals stimulating too many male hormones and makes the sebum production go crazy;

PCOS; and hyperandrogenism, which we will talk about in a later chapter.

There are some external factors as well that contribute to oily skin. Some people find their skin getting too oily because they wash their face too many times in a day! Yes, you read that right, and yes, you can go back, read that on repeat and drill that into your brain. I know it sounds counterintuitive, but you must understand that your skin is a magical self-balancing organ. When you wash your face too much, your skin responds by producing more sebum to balance the excessive dryness created by the extra washing. So, it eventually results in sebum production that just gets out of hand.

How much is too much? In my book, cleansing more than three times a day is too much. I have met patients who wash their face up to ten times a day because they simply hate the sensation of oil on their skin, and they actually have had the oiliest skin I've ever encountered. Once I got them to change their cleansing routines, their oiliness reduced significantly, and just with washing their face two to three times a day! I know it sounds crazy that it is that simple, but it is.

DR K'S PRO-TIP

For those of you who hate the greasy feeling but don't want to wash your face too much, use a biodegradable face wipe, a cotton gauze with saline water, cleanse with plain water, or just use a blotting paper to reduce some of that excess oil. I also sometimes add an afternoon peel pad with alpha hydroxy acids or salicylic acid in it for some extra skin clarifying.

REMEMBER!

Key oil-balancing ingredients to look for in your skincare:

- Salicylic acid 1-2 per cent, green tea 3 per cent, niacinamide 2 per cent for reducing the amount of oil secretion;

- Bentonite or fuller's earth or Moroccan clay for soaking up oil; and

- Vitamin A or retinol 0.5 per cent for reducing follicular obstruction (salicylic acid, too, can help reduce follicular obstruction, by the way).

Now, some specific products that are ideal for oily skin:

Cleanser: Look for a gentle cleanser designed to balance sebum production. Cleansers with zinc gluconate balance the amount of oil produced, while ingredients such as salicylic acid are ideal for cleansing within follicles where the gland that produces sebum exists. It also selectively cuts through that grease, and effectively reduces the amount of sebum made. It prevents obstruction of follicles by the sebum. Look for 1 per cent salicylic acid for more sensitive skin and 2 per cent salicylic acid for more resilient skin.

Avoid excessive foaming: more foam *does not* mean more clean. In fact, it can actually result in irritation of the skin. Ingredients such as sulphates can also result in skin irritation and barrier damage if the pH isn't balanced and if too much is used or left on for too long. So, the cleanser you use on your oily skin absolutely shouldn't over-foam.

Toner: I am not a huge believer in toners, but if you really must have one, you must avoid those with alcohol in them. Alcohol will dry out the skin excessively, resulting in the same thing that happens with over-washing: excess sebum production, thus worsening the condition of oily skin. Instead, for oily skin, look for ingredients such as salicylic acid, witch hazel, or green tea. Green tea has been known to reduce oil secretion, function well for anti-ageing, and help calm the skin.

MAKE YOUR OWN TONER

Make green tea with sterile or RO water. Put it in the fridge for an hour. Then put it into a spritz bottle and use as a toner!

You can mix it with a little khus water or coconut water for extra cooling benefits. Make this daily. Do not store because bacteria can grow really easily in water-based solutions that don't have preservatives in them.

Moisturizer: So here, it's up to you. If you are feeling greasy, you don't need a moisturizer. You are moist enough. Use one as an SOS, only if you feel dry. (If your skin is oily yet dehydrated, then the addition of a humectant-based moisturizer might be helpful, but we will discuss this when we talk about dehydrated skin shortly). Essentially, listen to your skin; don't just do what the marketing gurus tell you. If your skin feels like it has too many layers on it and you just feel too oily, your skin is telling you: 'Hey you don't need that moisturizer!'

Now, say you feel a little drier after cleansing and want to apply one, then look for a gel or light lotion-based moisturizer. Make sure it's heavy on the water, and with fewer oil components in it.

Typically, in the morning, when you are applying your sunblock, you may want to skip that moisturizer, but at night after any oil-reducing products, you may want to use one.

Normal skin

Technically, combination skin is normal skin, being 'normal' enough. And normal skin is the ideal. Few people have this. Genetically, we all have more oil glands in the T-zone, so we make more oil there naturally. People who somehow don't make more oil there, are the aberration. Normal skin is just good luck and good genes.

And if you have it, your only skincare guideline is: keep it really simple. You want to maintain the health of your skin. Avoid foaming cleansers – the more the foam, the more you dry out your skin, and the more it gets imbalanced and sensitive. All you have to do is moisturize well and wear sunblock.

Use actives (ingredients with high efficacy such as AHAs, retinol, peptides, and vitamin C) based on concern: ageing, pigmentation, glow. But don't overdo it – you want to keep your skin balanced because you are lucky enough to already have it balanced. So, you do less! Not more!

Combination skin: The real normal

There is nothing wrong with your combination skin, people! Your skin is normal. You are normal. Please don't buy into the marketing hype that this needs to be fixed. It's like the benchmarks they set for models: you can't be 5'11 and 110 pounds. (Please do not expect yourself to be the giraffe of skin.)

Skincare for combination skin is simple. Determine what time of day your skin feels most oily – morning or night. At that time, use a gentle foam-based cleanser or an anti-oil cleanser with salicylic acid/zinc/niacinamide/green tea once a day. For other times, non-foaming milk cleansers are fine.

Moisturize when you feel normal, skip the moisturizer when you feel greasy. Listen to your skin and go with what it tells you. Do what it needs. That's my mantra. That and: sunblock, sunblock, sunblock!

Dry skin

Red herring for those with dry skin: Foam is your enemy! It will dry you out. Products that will be your best friend if you have dry skin:

Cleanser: You need to be using cleansing milks and/or cleansing oils. If your skin is acne prone as well, use cleansing milks.

Moisturizer: Use moisturizers with ingredients such as ceramides, natural moisturizing agents (natural humectants already present in the skin, e.g. sodium lactate, lactic acid, urea), essential fatty acids (which are a part of the brick and mortar of the skin barrier). Basically, use heavy moisturizers and moisturize during the day again.

Healthy Vs Unhealthy Skin Barrier

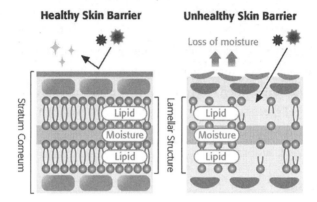

Sunblock: Must use as the sun dries you out even more.

Oils: At night after applying moisturizer, consider facial oils. If your dry skin is acne-prone too, grapeseed oil works well for it. If not, rosehip oil is my favourite.

Mask: You can always use a hydrating mask.

Facial Mists: These can be helpful underneath a moisturizer but alone, they can cause more dryness because they take water from inside the skin as they evaporate from its surface.

Sensitive skin

You can have oily, combination, normal or dry skin while being sensitive. Sensitive typically means your skin is easily irritated by-products, you get rashes easier, you may flush more, and you may get little bumps or even pimples from time to time. We typically call skin that has rosacea 'sensitive skin'. Rosacea is becoming increasingly common and often occurs at a younger age now, even though, typically, it is a genetic condition and found more in Caucasian skin. This is because of pollution, too much screen usage, and UV damage (the sun is more potent with less ozone, and even more so in India). Sometimes, your skincare routine can also contribute to rosacea, for example, scrubbing too much, excessive use of foaming washes, washing the face too much (which damages the skin barrier and makes it more sensitive), using pH imbalanced face washes, using too many acids and retinols throughout the day, getting facials too frequently (a facial a week is too much), and using topical steroids. I have seen many patients in India get skin-lightening products over the counter, which causes rosacea along with thin and sensitive skin.

DR K'S PRO-TIP

Keep it simple!

- Use simple skincare products that are artificial-fragrance-free, colour-free, foam-free. (These are the only 'frees' you need! Everything else can be managed.)

- Wear lots of sunblock.

- Use air filters at home.

- Cleanse your skin less.

- Do treatments/facials/home DIYs no more than once in a few weeks.

- Any AHAs/BHAs/retinols: Use these in limited percentages, building up over time.

- Do skin fasting: Once day a week or one week a month – only cleanse, moisturize and wear sunblock. No other products. You can even cleanse just with water for this.

Acne-prone skin

Any skin type, even sensitive skin, can be acne-prone. Acne-prone skin means your pores are likely to get obstructed and that your hormones make you more likely to get acne.

If you have acne-prone skin, Korean skincare is not for you. We are not Korean. Koreans have fewer oil glands, and their skin makes less oil; they don't usually get acne, like we do in India. K-beauty will not give you glass skin. K-beauty will drain your wallet and give you zits. Koreans are naturally pretty low on pores, and they also engage in heavy preventative skincare and therapies early on. Indian skin has more oil glands, creates more oil, and experiences a tougher, more pollution-heavy environment than Korean skin has to.

With acne-prone skin, it's important for you to do less and keep it simple. Your skincare routine should be three to four steps maximum. *Fewer layers, less obstruction* – that's your mantra!

In pandemic times, proper mask care is important for acne-prone skin. 'Maskne' is a real thing! Also called acne mechanica, masks can cause acne due to buildup of sweat, oil, obstruction, friction and constant pressure on the area. Use cotton masks or surgical masks and change them every 4 hours. For cotton masks, wash them after every use.

COMMON SKIN CONCERNS

Let's talk about some common issues I hear from my patients.

Acne

Nearly 80 per cent of people suffer from acne at least once in their lifetime, and it seems like it's plaguing people more and more these days. Now, adults are getting a lot more acne than before, as I often hear, 'I thought I grew out of this in my teenage years!' Among teenagers, acne has to do with the hormonal changes of pre-puberty and puberty; so yes, many teenagers do grow out of it. But if it is not treated, it can leave a lot of scars that can last for an entire lifetime. So, we prefer treating acne as soon as possible, usually with some lifestyle changes and medicated creams. Sometimes, we need oral medications, but that depends on how resistant the acne is. And, of course, if the acne is really tough to treat, we will check for PCOS as well. Also, we find that 30 per cent of acne in adults tends to be due to PCOS or some other hormonal condition, so the first thing I do is check how your hormones are doing.

The next, most common cause is incorrect product usage. And another one can be dandruff on the scalp or face, or rosacea that often looks like acne because it can have pimples too. Finally, face masks are increasingly becoming a reason for getting acne or 'maskne' in COVID times, as I talked about earlier. So, how we do our skincare now and manage our masks is quite crucial to maintaining good skin.

What does acne look like?

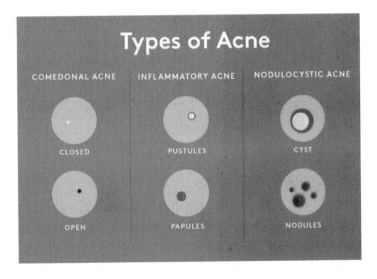

Comedonal acne refers to blackheads and whiteheads. At first, pores get obstructed by dead skin cells, oil and other detritus, and form what's called comedones. Then, these pores get infected with bacteria from the environment or with existing skin bacteria that results in inflammation, which then becomes inflammatory acne. The open comedones are blackheads and the closed ones are whiteheads. And those pesky little bumps under your skin are also comedones that are acne about to make an appearance in the future.

Inflammatory acne can either be small with pustules and papules, or large with nodulocystic acne. Basically, it means that there is a lot of inflammation happening around this follicular obstruction, so your white cells and immune system have been activated, resulting in swelling – that's why the red bumps! And remember, the more the inflammation, the more marks and scars happen, too.

Nodulocystic acne are deep acne nodules that are resistant to treatment. They typically need oral isotretinoin for resolution. Moreover, in the case of PCOS or hyperandrogenism, hormonal medications or anti-androgen medicines may be needed.

How to treat these different kinds of acne?

Comedonal acne typically needs salicylic acid cleansers to remove obstructions from the pores, and topical retinoids to increase epidermal desquamation (shedding) and get rid of acne under the skin. A purging process will occur for the first couple of months, but the acne that would have happened many months later then gets cleared out.

When it comes to pustular and papular acne, we typically need topical or oral antibiotics, which must be prescribed by an aesthetic doctor or a dermatologist.

Acne typically takes three to six months to go away, and I recommend slowly reducing the medications after that so the acne doesn't rebound. In hormonal conditions, I definitely recommend maintenance medications or creams so that the acne doesn't come back.

Acne scars

As if acne wasn't troubling enough, the dreaded skin condition can also lead to permanent scars on the skin. These range from shallow depressions scars to deep and narrow depressions of the skin. These depressions start off as bright pink purple, brown or red, but eventually settle into the colour of the skin and leave a crater-like effect. These flat shallow depressions are called atrophic scars and include boxcar scars, ice-pick scars, and rolling scars. In addition to this, the skin might also form keloid or hypertrophic scars that are created from skin tissue in a larger shape of the acne around the spots where it occurs.

Sometimes, acne can also cause post-inflammatory hyperpigmentation, i.e., dark or red spots on your skin where the pimple occurs.

I totally understand how traumatic acne scars can be. In terms of skincare, creams don't help much, but silicone gels can help hydrate the skin. Products with retinol help boost collagen. But to actually remove acne scars, you need treatments such as ablative lasers, fillers, and microneedling. As troubling as these scars may be, with the correct treatment, you *can* get rid of them!

Acne look-alikes

Many a time, your skin will erupt into acne-like formations. They look like acne but are something else. What can they be? Let's find out.

Rosacea, as we have already discussed, is a type of sensitive skin condition, but it's much worse than that. It can cause flushing, redness and a sensation of heat that occurs when triggered by exercise, heat, certain foods (discussed in our upcoming food chapter), alcohol and smoking. It can cause dilated or broken blood vessels. It can also cause sebaceous hyperplasia, where the oil glands increase in size and the nose can even become bigger due to it, while pores dilate. This is called rhinophyma. And finally, it can cause deep and painful pimples and also papules that can look like pimples.

The best ingredients for rosacea include azelaic acid, and some medicated creams that have ingredients such as ivermectin or pimecrolimus, which should be prescribed and monitored by a physician. And you must wait for a good twelve weeks for the full results. Often, your skin specialist will find that you have rosacea and acne at the same time and will treat both in the prescribed regimen. This is why you really do need a good doctor.

Seborrheic dermatitis happens when dandruff or oil on the scalp triggers pimples and papules around the nose and T-zone area. Sometimes, this also manifests as oiliness or scaling around the nose and T-zone. This is due to sensitivity to a yeast, called

Malassezia furfur, which is naturally present in the skin. This is ideally treated with a good dandruff shampoo and an anti-fungal cream that is prescribed by your doctor. Again, all these conditions can occur simultaneously, so consulting your doctor is a must!

Pores are something everyone has, and one cannot really get rid of them. They get dilated because of repeated obstruction and oil secretion. They also get bigger due to ageing. So, how can you deal? I suggest: reduce oil secretion, follow the oily skin rules, and use products that have ingredients suitable for your skin type.

Add anti-ageing ingredients, such as retinol, peptides or bakuchiol, to your routine so that you can boost collagen and keep the skin tighter. Treatment wise, I think microneedling helps boost baby collagen (the same collagen you had as a baby) and helps reduce pore size over time. Laser rejuvenation also helps boost collagen and tightens pores. Regular skin maintenance is needed to prevent pores from becoming enlarged; this is achieved with an active skincare routine and a good monthly facial regimen.

Complexion

This is something many people come to me for, asking me how to 'improve' it. Complexion is genetic. The colour is genetic. Accept your natural colour, please. It is what makes you beautiful! All those skin-whitening and bleaching creams are bad and damaging for your skin. They make it irritated and sensitive, and will cause rosacea and prove to be problematic over time.

One of the most common complaints I hear is that 'my face is darker than my body'. This happens because of cumulative sun exposure, pigmentation, and tanning – all these can cause this difference in complexion. Low levels of antioxidants in the body can also be a factor.

If this is your complaint, add glutathione, vitamin C and NAC supplements to your routine to boost antioxidant levels. Do run these supplements by your doctor though, because if you have allergies to certain medications or if you have liver issues, then these meds may not be right for you. Also, use sunblock: two-finger length, every four hours indoors or outdoors (yes, exposure to sunlight and blue light happens indoors as well). And trust me, I am not crazy when I say this. Sunblock is a barrier and there needs to be enough on your face to create a shield against the sun. Every time I tell my patients, they look at me like I have grown three horns on my head. I promise it will be absorbed into the skin. It will take time, which is why it is good to apply sunscreen at least thirty minutes before you leave home. But your skin will thank me and hopefully you will too.

AHAs, vitamin C, arbutin, kojic acid, and liquorice acid are great ingredients to use at night to improve complexion variations.

If you're looking for treatments, here are the ones I suggest:

1. Peels: Effective, but short term. Too many might make the skin too thin, so please make use of them in a balanced way.

2. Microdermabrasion: Removing dead damaged skin is an effective way to get rid of dull, tanned skin. Minimal side effects and quick results.

3. LED: Low-level red and yellow light therapy add a lit-from-within glow, but usually with a lot of sittings and often in addition to another therapy. I try to add on LED to a lot of my treatments to calm skin and add an extra collagen boost.

4. Microneedling: This improves skin signalling to prevent excess discolouration from outside trauma such as pollution, sun, and stress. It helps boost baby collagen and reverses ageing, making skin healthier and younger. Your skin is more toned, and both the texture and complexion improve.

5. Laser Toning: Laser toning is designed to reduce pigmentation, improve pores, and improve the clarity of the skin. It should be done on a regular basis to keep improving and maintaining the skin simultaneously. Typically, laser toning uses lasers based on a Q-switched technology. There are thousands of different types of Q-switched lasers, but not all Q-switched lasers are the same. Different countries, different energies, different regulations, different methods of energy delivery – please don't assume Q-switch is one-size-fits-all. The machines matter and the operator matters. How someone uses their machine is *vital*. Expertise is everything.

6. Picosure Laser: This is the fastest and most effective in improving complexion discolouration and any

form of pigmentation. It is well known as the most powerful laser in the world for pigmentation and tattoo removal. It may be more expensive, but the results speak for themselves.

Wrinkles and ageing

Ageing shows up on every skin layer. About 70 per cent of ageing is from the sun. Your top epidermis layer gets weaker and drier as you age. Your dermis shows more pigmentation and freckles. And your third layer, the hypodermis, sees lower levels of collagen and elastin, causing wrinkles and sagging.

How to treat it? Use skincare products with ingredients that boost collagen (e.g. vitamin C, retinol, bakuchiol, peptides), ingredients that increase cell turnover (e.g. AHAs), and ingredients that prevent ageing and damage from pollution and sun (e.g. vitamin C/ferulic acid).

In terms of treatments, I usually recommend:

1. Botox/fillers/PRP/skin boosters
2. Non-invasive tightening such as Ultherapy and Thermage or radiofrequency technologies
3. Laser rejuvenation or ablative resurfacing
4. Microneedling (notice how microneedling is everywhere?)

Pigmentation

Pigmentation is a common concern amongst my clients, probably because Indian skin is extremely susceptible to hyper-pigmentation. Four out of five people suffer from it. In a majority of the cases, the main cause of pigmentation and ageing is sun exposure. Other factors that influence it are genes, pollution, wrong skincare products, hair colour, and hormones: any or all of these can cause pigmentation.

Did you know that 70 per cent of Indian women suffer from pigmentation on their forehead and around their mouth? Termed AIPFP, or Acquired Idiopathic Patterned Facial Pigmentation, this condition affects many people in this particular geographic latitude. It's annoying, but it's very common and most people struggle with it. The good news is that it is also very treatable. PDL (Pigmentary Demarcation Lines) are sharply demarcated patches that can occur around the mouth, the eyes, and other areas, and are also pretty common. Natural dyschromia is a simple description of pigmentation common in older clients, where cumulative skin damage results in dark pigmentation on the forehead and next to the eyes and cheek (malar areas).

A less common pigmentation disorder is *melasma*, which is characterized by patches on the cheeks, upper lip, nose, jawline and/or forehead. Not all of these areas need to be affected for it to be melasma. It's usually associated with both sun exposure and hormones, so many women experience it after taking oral contraceptives or during pregnancy. Often, removing the hormonal-inciting factor helps, but not always, in which case treatments and skincare are necessary. It is important to understand melasma because it's more chronic and can flare up due to stress, weather changes, sun exposure or hormonal changes.

And finally, pigmentation doesn't spare the body either. Another condition called cutaneous macular amyloidosis is commonly found in Indian women and is characterized by slate-grey, dark bluish-black discolouration on the back and/or arms. It's worse in areas that are regularly scratched. This is tougher to treat and, almost always, requires treatments because creams can't target the cause so well.

The most important advice I give for all types of pigmentation is sun protection. Indoor lighting and screens can cause pigmentation as well. Sunblock really is your best friend.

In skincare, I recommend you use products with preventative ingredients such as vitamin C, ferulic acid or arbutin, alpha arbutin, AHAs, liquorice extract, kojic acid, cysteamine, salicylic acid, retinol; all of these help prevent and treat pigmentation. I vote against skin-lightening creams, unless overseen by a skin doctor as they are known to cause irritation and sensitivity and, in rare instances, they can cause something called ochronosis, a slate-grey discolouration that occurs due to an ingredient called hydroquinone. They can also cause rosacea and skin thinning. However, they can be used to treat discolouration under the advice of your skin doctor.

In terms of treatments, lasers, peels and microneedling are often necessary and work effectively.

Under-eye circles

Let's face it, dark circles, a.k.a those pesky, black circles around the eyes, only look cute on pandas. In the case of humans, they make our eyes look puffed, pull down our look, and attract frustrating comments like 'Did you sleep last night?' And it's no surprise that so many of you come to me with this complaint.

Under-eye circles are of four types:

1. There are those caused by discolouration or pigmentation, which can be triggered by sun damage, genes or ageing.

2. Another kind is hollow, recessed eyes. These are mostly an effect of genetics or ageing.

3. Under-eye bags are also a common issue. These happen when collagen weakens and fat bags that live under the skin herniate out.

4. Dark circles can also be a vascular issue. These can happen due to less sleep and thin skin. In this kind, you can see the blood vessels. Fluid can accumulate due to low lymphatic drainage, causing under-eye swelling.

I will talk about under-eye skincare in detail later on. But in a nutshell, I'd suggest you look for vitamin C, arbutin and kojic/liquorice extract for pigmentation. Use hesperidin, Vitamin K or caffeine, for the vascular kind of under-eye circles. You should use retinol, peptides, bakuchiol for ageing and collagen boosting. These creams, however, are more of a preventative measure. If you already have under-eye circles, treatments are necessary.

For hollows and bags, I suggest fillers, Ulthera, or surgery. Radiofrequency can also help, but you'd need eight or more sessions for it to show results. For discolouration and wrinkles, the best way to go is laser rejuvenation and microneedling.

3

HAIR'S TO YOU

ALL ABOUT YOUR MANE

O fleece, that down the neck waves to the nape!
O curls! O perfume nonchalant and rare!
O ecstasy! To fill this alcove shape
With memories that in these tresses sleep,
I would shake them like penions in the air!

– 'Her Hair', Charles Baudelaire

Hair makes us feel beautiful. It can make or break a perfect outfit. A good hair day is our mood-lifter. We spend remarkable amounts of time and money on getting our hair to look a certain way. We colour, groom, highlight, change textures, take treatments just to be able to wear that head of hair like a crown. We do so much, but the results rarely match our efforts. Let me tell you that all of it is temporary, and some of it can even cause long-term damage.

I know what you're thinking. How can my hair look better? Thicker? More voluminous? Shinier? Less frizzy? How can it grow longer? To what extent do I trust my beauty parlour lady? Why does she keep telling me to do a keratin treatment for every hair problem I have? Do hair spas really work? Which shampoo is the best? How often do I wash it? Why is my hair falling out?

This is the running commentary I hear from my clients when they walk through the door. Curly, straight, thick, thin, long, short – hair is an all-time hot topic with everyone. So many questions, so much anxiety (which, ironically, may cause more hair fall!)

But don't worry, I am here to calm your nerves with real, honest information and solutions!

Listening to my clients, the one question I arrived at was if we truly know our hair. Most of us don't. The first step to haircare is to understand it inside out.

Let's start with types of hair. When we think hair, we think: thick, thin, curly, straight, frizzy, soft, long, short. But contrary to popular categorization, hair is essentially of two kinds: porous and non-porous.

TYPES OF HAIR

Porous hair is the type of hair in which the hair cuticle is damaged/lifted and moisture, products, and oils pass through it easily. This type of hair often tends to tangle and get frizzy. It is usually caused by hair colouring, treatments, and poor haircare.[1]

Non-porous hair is the type where the cuticle is firmly in place and, therefore, it is healthy and shiny. It tends to repel water and doesn't absorb products easily. It is prone to build-up because products sit on the surface of the hair instead of passing through it.

Do you sometimes wish that you had the kind of hair that you had as a child? That was actually non-porous hair. But as we age, all hair will gain some porosity. Low, medium and high porosity is how we would gauge the porosity level of your hair. And the more porous it is, the more quickly it absorbs water from the air, the more your hair fluffs up until you get FRIZZ! We will talk about frizz in a bit.

First, let's check what type of hair you have? Porous or non-porous? Your hair can have varying degrees of porosity. Here are two simple, fun ways to find out how porous (or non-porous) your hair is:

The Float Test: Take a couple of strands of hair from your comb and drop them into a bowl of water. Let them sit for two to four minutes. If your hair floats, you have low porosity. However, if it sinks, you have high porosity.

The Slip 'n' Slide Test: Take a strand of hair and slide your fingers up the shaft (toward the scalp). If you feel little bumps along the way, it means that your hair cuticle is lifted and you have high porosity. If your fingers slip smoothly, then you have low porosity hair.

The other categorizations of hair are mostly based on genetics. Whether hair is curly, wavy, or straight depends on genes, as does the length of your hair. The porosity of hair, too, depends on genes but there are a number of habits and practices that can affect it, which includes shampooing too frequently, wet combing or brushing, touching your hair too much, treatments that change the bonds of the hair (rebounding, keratin, straightening, perming, colouring).

Any treatment that changes the pH of the hair will also make your hair more porous. Now, what is the pH of hair?

This is where we get a bit technical. pH stands for 'potential of hydrogen'. It is the measure of the acidity or basicity of any solution or substance. When the concentration of hydrogen ions is lower, the pH is higher, and the higher the pH, the lesser the acidity. A pH of 7 in any solution is considered neutral. When the pH drops below 7, the solution begins to get acidic. Any value higher than 7, and it acquires a basic nature.

The pH is also measured for skin and hair. A healthy pH value of the scalp is between 4.5 and 5.5, as this is optimal to prevent infections and breakouts. The pH of hair should stay between 4.5 and 7 or you risk causing damage to it. Non-porous hair can handle pH variation better than porous hair, but it is still better to maintain the pH within range. When pH is outside the limits of 4.5 and 7, hair is far more vulnerable to damage because the scalp may get inflamed and take the acid or base (alkali) into the hair, beneath the cuticle, and this can damage the proteins of your hair. It certainly strips some oils from the hair.

What is pH?

The **pH scale** is a measure of how **acidic** or **basic** a solution is.

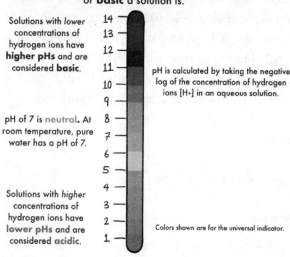

Solutions with *lower* concentrations of hydrogen ions have **higher pHs** and are considered **basic**.

pH is calculated by taking the negative log of the concentration of hydrogen ions [H+] in an aqueous solution.

pH of 7 is neutral. At room temperature, pure water has a pH of 7.

Solutions with *higher* concentrations of hydrogen ions have **lower pHs** and are considered acidic.

Colors shown are for the universal indicator.

Most hair can withstand extremely low or high pH values for brief exposures. But if your hair has been bleached, damaged or is otherwise vulnerable, even brief exposures to pH extremes can have lasting effects. Where would you encounter such exposures? Hair treatments such as keratin have a pH of 2.8, which is extremely low. But hair relaxing (chemical straightening) and hair perming rely on highly alkaline (high pH) solutions to achieve their objective and are not good for the health of your hair. I often have clients with severe hair-fall post keratin hair straightening or perms because their hair strands are irreversibly damaged. The hair ends up getting tangled easily and breaking frequently.

You can easily find out the pH of any solution you are using on your hair by buying pH strips. If the pH of the solution you're using is too high or too low, it may not be good for your hair. Fun fact: most shampoos that claim to be all-natural actually have a higher than needed pH.[2]

So, for hair, I'd say: keep it simple. It's cool to have fun with your hair, but first gauge your hair type. *Know your hair.* If your hair is already too porous or damaged, hair keratin or perm treatments will worsen it, sometimes permanently.

Now, let's talk about some common hair issues that everyone faces.

COMMON HAIR ISSUES

Hair frizz

Are you someone who detests monsoons or humidity because your hair suddenly becomes uncomfortably large and no amount of taming efforts work long enough? Yes, your hair just got the frizz! What is frizzy hair? We talked about hair cuticles when we were discussing hair types. Frizz is basically hair with raised hair cuticles. Curly hair, damaged hair, coloured and treated hair – all have raised cuticles on the hair shaft, which are flat in normal hair. The cuticle is raised because it is dehydrated, so it takes up water from the humidity in the air and makes the hair 'full' or 'bloated', causing frizz.

How do you fix it? First, we flatten the cuticle by reducing hair treatments and colouring, all of which damage your hair cuticle. Reduce the frequency of shampooing! Your hair isn't as dirty as you think it is. Shampooing can strip the hair of its natural sebum (oil) when done too much or too often. When you shampoo, try to use either cold or lukewarm water because hot water also raises the cuticle. You can use acidic rinses, such as diluted apple cider vinegar or flat beer/champagne, to flatten the cuticle, although these will, at best, give you temporary results. The true key to reducing your frizz is to hydrate the cuticle![3]

DR K'S PRO-TIP

Here are some more hot tips to hydrate the cuticle and fight the frizz:

1. **Rinse** with saline water, which helps bind water into the strands.

2. Go **No Poo.** Reduce shampooing to one to two times a week. That way, you won't strip the hair of its natural oil. Also, shampoo only your scalp; the suds will clean the strands.

3. Wear **sunscreen or hairscreen** on your hair, so that the sun doesn't dry out the hair cuticle.

4. **Condition** the strands both before and after shampooing to protect from hair stripping.

5. **Oil** your hair with coconut oil.

6. Don't rely on anti-frizz **serums**, as their result is temporary. In fact, they often contain silicone, which may cause scalp build-up! I prefer to rub a little coconut oil as a natural serum.

How do you oil?[4]

Oiling can prove very useful in conditioning raised hair cuticles and resolving hair frizz. When you choose an oil, look at the percentage of lipids or fats, amount of penetrating triglycerides and the research. The data resoundingly says that the best oil to use is coconut oil. You can keep it on for two to twelve hours, with your hair wrapped in a heated towel.

What about the other oils? Coconut oil has enough triglyceride fats, which are the right size to be absorbed into the shaft, so it works best. Here are some other oils, with their different penetration ratios.

Oils with high penetration[5]	Percentage of oil that cuticles can absorb	Heat helps improve penetration	Hair penetration documented by research
Coconut oil	95%	Yes	Yes, excellent
Sunflower oil	91%	Yes	Yes
Castor oil	15%	Unknown	Not documented. Chemical structure not ideal for penetration but possible.
Olive oil	94%	Possible	Yes, good

Mustard seed oil	44.9%	Unknown	Not documented
Sweet almond oil	~99%	Unknown	Not documented
Apricot kernel oil	~100%	Unknown	Not documented
Argan oil	98%	Unknown	Not documented
Sesame seed oil	~86%	Unknown	Not documented
Grapeseed oil	99%	Unknown	Not documented
Rosehip oil	~97%	Unknown	Not documented
Flax seed (linseed) oil	99%	Unknown	Not documented
Cocoa butter	~98%	Unknown	Not documented
Oils with little to no hair penetration	**% Oil that cuticles can absorb**	**Penetration improves with heat?**	**Hair penetration documented by research**
Mineral oil			No penetration
Jojoba oil	less than 1%		No penetration

Hair loss (or Alopecia)

I know hair fall causes a lot of distress: you won't find a person who doesn't freak out from hair fall. When you see those clumps entangled in your comb or on the floor of your bathroom, you panic and it's understandable. But guess what? Most hair fall is manageable!

Let's talk about the most common form of it. The technical term for it is *Telogen Effluvium*, and it is totally normal to experience some hair fall now and then. Our hair, while we love it, is actually not needed for our bodies to function. So, when we go through the slightest of traumas (mild sickness, pregnancies, change of season – all traumas for our bodies), our body will go into 'survival-first' mode and put all its focus on the most important things, and then send the signal of what it is doing through our hair or skin.

On a healthy scalp, about 90 per cent of hair follicles are actively growing hair (this is called anagen hair) and about 9 per cent are inactive or resting hair (called telogen hair). Usually, a hair follicle actively grows an anagen hair for 3-5 years and then rests that hair for about 2-4 months (as telogen). When the hair follicle begins to push out a new anagen hair, it does so under an existing telogen or resting hair. Then[6] as this new hair begins to grow, it pushes out the telogen hair it is resting under and that is what we see on our combs, showers and pillows! It is totally normal to lose up to a hundred strands of hair in a day: it's all a part of our healthy hair cycle. Stress is not good for your hair; it causes more hair fall. It releases the hormones cortisone and cortisol in our bodies, and the latter directly impacts the hair follicles by inhibiting hair growth. So, take a deep breath and relax! Manage stress and keep that cortisol under control: the less you stress, the more your hair grows! Yay!

But sometimes, you will find that you're losing more than the normal amount of hair. Is there a reason to panic? Probably not. First, ask yourself – has your body recently been through any shock? In the case of a 'shock to your system', as much as 70 per cent of your anagen or active hair can be converted into telogen, which is what you see as that massive hair fall.

Some of the common triggers for hair loss:

- Childbirth: Postpartum hair loss. Giving birth is a massive change for the system and can cause hair fall. This can resolve after a few months or transition into female pattern alopecia (which, too, is treatable)

- Physiological neonatal hair loss: It's not just you, your baby is also losing hair. A newborn sheds a lot of hair, and it is completely normal (new moms, don't panic)

- Acute or chronic illness, especially if there is fever

- Surgical operation

- Accident

- Psychological stress

- Weight loss, unusual diet, or nutritional deficiency (e.g. iron deficiency)

- Certain medications
- Hormone issues such as thyroid
- Discontinuing contraceptive pills
- Overseas travel resulting in jetlag
- Skin disease affecting the scalp
- Excessive sun exposure
- COVID!

If you have gone through any of these experiences, I recommend first getting your blood tests done. Check your **ferritin** level: it should be above seventy for healthy hair growth (even though your body can function with lower levels of this). In case it is lower than seventy, you can treat it with iron supplements: take ferrous fumarate or ferrous sulphate (twice a day, 325 mg). Take it with vitamin C to improve absorption. In case you have a sensitive stomach, you can replace this with Ferrous Bi-glycinate. If you have thalessia or an iron-processing blood disorder, you are not a candidate for this vitamin. As a practice, always consult your doctor before taking any supplements. You should also keep your **vitamin B12** levels above 400 and **zinc** above seventy. And, check your **folic acid** and **vitamin D** levels. Getting your **thyroid** tested is also important in case of hair loss, as thyroid issues often affect hair. Diet-wise, I'd recommend focusing on foods with high biotin content and protein. But no whey or casein protein powders! In my experience, I have seen worsening of hair fall with these supplements.

Male Pattern and Female Pattern Baldness

Mostly, hair fall is manageable with the correct diagnosis at the correct time, but sometimes, it advances to male and female pattern baldness. And these days, pattern balding is increasingly being seen in younger people. Balding patterns are partially genetic and hereditary, but are often worsened by foods such as whey protein, dairy and sugar. Additionally, physiological conditions such as PCOS, hyperandrogenemia (excess male hormones) and even stress can contribute to it. Vitamin deficiencies will reveal it sooner. To manage hair fall, it is important to keep our health in check and avoid stress. Because stress causes hair fall, which causes more stress, which causes more hair fall! It's a vicious circle.

~

Did you know even men can get a version of PCOS that shows up as early balding and insulin resistance? So, if you are a man and balding in your early thirties, or even before that, it's time to get a full enhanced insulin and blood sugar profile done, and start working on your diet; check out the food chapter coming up.

For severe hair loss and balding, I usually prescribe minoxidil. It is a hair growth medicine that needs to be applied to the scalp, and I think it is the gold standard for hair growth. It does take about three to six months to show results and, initially, causes some temporary hair loss. But that involves the dead hair that would fall off anyway. It can cause some scalp irritation too. When you stop its usage, some of the newly grown hair can fall off again, but not all will (in most cases). It is something that you can even continue using long term. Side effects are rare; in some cases, it may cause issues with libido and some minor individual side effects. Sometimes, dandruff and scalp sensitivity may occur and, paradoxically, more facial hair growth may be observed. But they are rare. RARE! Don't let the fear of a rare side effect keep you from ensuring healthy hair growth! If it doesn't work, you can stop it. Important note though, not everyone can tolerate minoxidil, and it has to be used properly and monitored for the best results in consultation with a doctor. Please don't go buying minoxidil without talking to your skin witch!

Another conversation that comes up with my clients is that around **hair transplant**. My advice on that is to delay it as much as possible, because after some time, it will need to be repeated. I'd say, first go for everything preventive and non-invasive and manage for as long as you can, until you absolutely cannot, and only then go in for a transplant.

Dandruff

Dandruff is not a fun problem to have. It is caused by seborrheic dermatitis. Basically, it is a sensitivity to yeast, called *Malassezia furfur*, on the scalp and can occur episodically, especially if there are weather changes around you or if you change your hair products. Sometimes, drying out of the scalp from excessive shampooing can also cause it. Medications such Minoxidil can trigger it as well. The line of treatment I recommend for dandruff is using a proper medicated shampoo and avoiding oiling the scalp. It does need preventive care as well, such as consuming less sugar, less dairy, fewer artificial and processed foods. You should also avoid hair products such as pomades, waxes and serums, as the build-up from them will worsen dandruff. Be very careful with the shampoos and products you choose. Use anti-dandruff shampoo once a week or once in two weeks when the dandruff resolves. Take extra care of your hair during weather changes. Pollution can also trigger dandruff, so be careful when the AQI rises up!

HAIR DYES AND COLOURS

Client: Dr K, can I get my hair dyed?
Dr K: No!

I know it looks fun, but I would mostly discourage chemical hair colouring. Hair dyes with PPD or PPT are can cause severe allergic rashes, swelling, and irritation of the scalp. They also make you more sensitive to the sun and can even cause pigmentation in your surrounding skin, which can be permanent. These reactions can happen even years after using hair colours. It is best to use natural hair colours such as indigo and henna (but even then, watch out for the ones that say 'long lasting' as they may have PPD in them!) However, if you absolutely must use a PPD hair colour, then try to use as little as you can. Reduce the frequency. Here, even I am a hypocrite because, while I try to use natural hair colours, sometimes if I am in a rush, I will use a regular PPD-based hair colour to cover up those greys.

NOTE: Some people are allergic to henna or indigo, so even natural hair dyes are not without risk. However, a PPD allergy is way more severe than an indigo allergy.

DR K'S PRO-TIP

While using PPD colour, put vaseline on the skin around your head that may come in contact with the colour (skin on your forehead, ears, etc.), and avoid the sun for the next seven days to minimize the risk of pigmentation in the skin.

BIOTIN & HAIR SUPPLEMENTS

For biotin to work, you need to take it in the right dose, which is not available anywhere. Most places stock a dosage size of 5 mg, which is ineffective, the majority of hair supplements and hair gummies sold in medicine stores are simply marketing gimmicks. They have ineffective doses of any requisite vitamins. I believe in targeting the actual source of the deficiency and treating that. Although I have found that collagen supplements are usually helpful and so are some cyclical nutritional therapy supplements, these are adjuncts, and not the main event. The vitamin deficiency or the cause needs to be treated, everything else is EXTRA!

MYTHBUSTER	
Popular beliefs	**Marketing claims you should ignore**
Keratin straightening will prevent hair fall – **False**	More foam – More cleansing
Shedding season – **True**	Soap-based shampoos – High pH. Worsen hair damage
Water change causes hair fall – **True**	
Shampooing every day is necessary – **False**	All natural – Often means pH is very high and can cause more hair damage
Oiling for Dandruff – **False** (makes it worse actually)	Dry shampoo is safe
Sulphate-free means it's safe – **False**	Sulphate-free – There are lots of detergents that are irritating, not just sulphates
Stress can make you grey – **False**	
Keeping hair in a braid overnight is good for your hair – **True**	

DR K'S PRO-TIP[7]

- Avoid high-foam shampoos.

- Condition your strands before and after you shampoo your scalp. Don't use conditioner on your scalp! You shampoo the scalp and you condition your strands.

- Start collagen supplementation.

- Saline rinse for quick DIY no-frizz.

- Don't pull your hair back too tightly, as it causes hair thinning.

- Use a silk pillowcase.

- Avoid blow-drying your hair or getting too many blowouts and curling treatment.

- Do not wet comb.

- Keratin treatments and perming can cause hair fall, so, avoid them too.

- Hair highlights can also cause breakage, so reduce the frequency and practise good hair practices with gentle shampoos and good conditioning between highlighting.

NAILS

Did you know that your nails are made of the same stuff as your hair? It's totally true, and the stuff is called keratin. Nails continually grow throughout life due to the action of the matrix, which is connected to blood vessels. Evolutionarily, nails were probably developed in humans to help them forage for food, climb trees, and to improve and protect our touch nerve receptors, which are plentiful at the tips of our digits.

Over time, we have devised ways to take care of our nails and ensure their wellbeing. But, manicures, too, can cause nail issues. Artificial nails can leave your nails brittle, parched and dry. To apply false nails on your nails, you have to make the surface rough, and you have to use chemicals to apply and acetone to remove them.[8] This process weakens nails and can result in long-term nail damage. Soak-off gel nails are easier on the nails, but can still be a problem if used repetitively.[9]

Tips for good nail care:

- Use artificial nails sparingly.
- Take nail polish holidays for a week or two so the nails can repair themselves.
- Don't cut your cuticles at the salon to prevent infections.
- Apply Vaseline jelly to the nails and cuticles regularly to help them repair and prevent further damage.

4

JUST LIKE GRANDMA USED TO SAY

HOW EFFECTIVE IS YOUR HOME-MADE SKINCARE?

Client: Dr K, my skin is getting dry and irritated for no reason! I haven't changed my routine at all. Why?

Dr K: You haven't used anything else on your skin?

Client: Only natural stuff, like walnut powder and sandalwood scrubs every day.

Dr K: !!!!!

India has a beautiful tradition of making things work with whatever is available. This aspect, often called 'jugaad', is proof of Indian ingenuity and creativity, and I love it. Except when you apply it to your skin!

Grandma's secrets, home-made skincare, DIY (do-it-yourself) products are hardly ever a solution and certainly never a long-term solution for your skin. Many a time, they end up causing more harm than good and, sometimes, even irreversible damage. If you have absolutely normal and great skin, then sure, using yoghurt or fruit on your face will be okay. The reason for this is not the home-made product you are using but the fact that your skin is already great and the few actives present in the fruit or yoghurt or DIY solution helps maintain it. With naturally great skin, it is not the home-made solution you are using, but your skin itself that requires little maintenance. The good thing about 'natural' or home-made solutions is that, unless you are trying a new DIY solution every day, they don't usually irritate your skin too much. And the usual yoghurt, fruit combinations (except for lemon) are pretty gentle when used once a week. So, with already good skin, you are not excessively using active products but only applying those that boost it gently and just enough to maintain that skin health.

For a gentle boost that is temporary, a safe home remedy can be nice. But remember, not all home remedies suit everyone, and you can still get irritated by a DIY. Most home remedies may make you sensitive to the sun, so be aggressive with your sun protection. Further, check with your skin or hair doc if you can do the home remedies mentioned and how to alter your skincare or haircare routine, treatment regimen, hair removal or bleaching routine to accommodate the DIY.

HOME REMEDIES THAT WORK WONDERS

For acne and zits, use warm compress for a few minutes a few times a day brings out the pus from underneath the skin.

- Ice will reduce the redness, so you can use an ice cube on the zit.

- Tea tree oil[10] has been shown to reduce acne lesions by 25–60 per cent if you use it for twelve weeks. Note that it's not curative, but now that all the topical antibiotics are there, having an alternative antibacterial option that doesn't have resistance is great![11]

- Sulfur is great for its anti-bacterial properties. Use Mario Badescu's drying lotion, which has sulphur and works wonders due to its antibacterial and anti-inflammatory effects.

For hair

- Apple cider vinegar (diluted) and beer hair rinse for softer, shinier and lustrous hair.

- For dry and frizzy hair, mix avocado and one egg with a little coconut oil. Apply the mix and let it dry, then wash off. Your hair will be much smoother and softer.

- Mix onion juice with some black tea and a drop or two of peppermint oil. Apply twice a week to encourage hair growth. Onion juice has been proven to reduce alopecia areata and increase hair growth. Black tea has caffeine, which is also shown to increase hair growth, while peppermint oil has menthol, which can be stimulatory.

For eyes

- Rest cold cucumber slices on your eyelids for five to ten minutes for an instantly refreshed look.
- Apply cold and refrigerated green tea bags on the eyes for five to ten minutes. Caffeine in the green tea constricts blood vessels, reduces vascular inflammation (so, it's great for those who look tired and puffy in the mornings) and reduces inflammation. The cold also vasoconstricts the blood vessels.[12]

For skin

GLOW BOOSTER

Ingredients:

Yoghurt or buttermilk, ½ tsp.

Tomato juice, ½ tsp.

Honey, ½ tsp.

Plum, enough for a pulpy texture, ½ or 1 whole

Method:

Once you apply the mask, gently rub using circular motions to exfoliate the skin. The ingredients contain a host of natural acids – from AHAs to glycolic acids – which work to get rid of rough, lacklustre cells and small bumps to give you super-smooth, tight skin.

AHAs, like glycolic and lactic acid, are well-known dermatology ingredients we use to treat pigmentation and enhance the glow. They are also present in chemical peels. Foods such as buttermilk, yoghurt, certain fruits and sugar also contain AHAs but in extremely low percentages.

APPLY ONCE A WEEK and avoid the sun for seven days and any strong actives the day before and the day after. Avoid bleach, as well.

GLOW MASK

Ingredients:

Yoghurt, ½ tbsp.

Honey, ½ tsp.

Amla powder, 1 tsp.

Room temperature water to mix for a thick consistency

Method:

Mix all the ingredients and keep on the face for five minutes, then wash it with lukewarm water. Amla powder contains a very high amount of vitamin C, which enhances glow and resolves pigmentation. However, I personally prefer products with high-quality vitamin C, because vitamin C gets inactivated very quickly when it's exposed to air. So, you want a stabilized form of vitamin C for it to have the desired effect.

DIY LACTIC ACID MASK (for dry, dull skin and under-eye rejuvenation)

Ingredients:

Honey, ½ tsp.

Yoghurt or buttermilk, ½ tsp.

Water, 2 tbsp.

Method:

Mix them all together and make a paste. Apply this mixture on the face evenly and under the eyes. Keep it for five minutes and rinse.

APPLY ONCE A WEEK and avoid the sun for seven days and any strong actives the day before, of and the day after. Avoid bleach as well.

ANTI-ACNE MASK (for clogged pores and acne-prone oily skin)

Ingredients:

Mint, ¼ cup

Grapeseed oil, ½ cup

Cabbage, ½ cup

Buttermilk, enough to make a thick paste

Method:

Wash mint leaves, crush them, and put them in a glass jar. Add grapeseed oil to the mix and let it sit for forty-eight hours. Mix soaked cabbage and buttermilk to create a thick paste, and then apply to the face. Watch out, it may feel irritating, and not all people can handle mint extract on their face without irritation.

Use this no more than once every two weeks and avoid the sun for seven days. Also avoid any strong actives the day before and the day after. Avoid bleach as well.

ICE CUBES

For instant pore minimizing, zit zapping and redness reduction, rub an ice cube all over your face for a minute. For an extra glow, freeze fresh orange juice into ice cubes. You will get some much-needed vitamin C.

PEELING AND SUNBURN RECIPE

Ingredients:

Aloe vera gel

Vaseline petroleum jelly

Method:

Mix equal parts cold aloe vera gel and Vaseline petroleum jelly, and apply it throughout the day on sunburnt skin.

Aloe vera is a wonderful calming and soothing ingredient. But it can often be used incorrectly. Due to its watery nature, it can also cause dryness and irritation when used without a moisturizer. In fact, some people are even allergic or sensitive to it. So please don't assume aloe vera is always right for you.

ALOE VERA

Perhaps the best-known botanical anti-inflammatory agent, aloe vera is popularly used to soothe both UV- and heat-induced burns. Made primarily of water (99.5 per cent), the colourless gel released from plant leaves contains a complex mixture of mucopolysaccharides, amino acids, and minerals. Several distinct compounds have been isolated from aloe-vera juice, including aletinic acid, aloe-emodin, aloin and choline salicylate. To confer anti-inflammatory effect, estimates suggest that the concentration of aloe vera must be at least 10 per cent. It's important to note that most skincare products use the powder form of aloe vera, which may not be equivalent to the fluid extracted from the plant's leaf.

NATURAL TONER

Ingredients:

Green tea

Water

Method:

Boil green tea in water and cool the mixture. Spritz this on your face twice a day for tighter pores and refreshed skin. It reduces oil secretion, prevents rosacea and has a calming effect.

Make it fresh daily because there is no preservative in a home DIY, and you certainly don't want to have bacterially contaminated DIYs.

For lips

Honey is the best ingredient used to moisturize your lips. With a little bit of care, you can achieve pink, luscious and soft lips, as you always wanted.

Mix brown sugar, honey and olive oil together and use it as a scrub for your lips. Honey is antiseptic and moisturizing, brown sugar is exfoliating and hydrating, while olive oil has healthy essential fatty acids for emollience.

LIP BRIGHTENER

Ingredients:

Pomegranate seeds, ¼ cup

Grated beetroot, ½ cup

Ghee, 1 tsp.

Method:

Crush and strain the pomegranate seeds. Retain the juice. Squeeze the beetroot and strain out the beetroot juice. Mix the pomegranate juice, beetroot juice and ghee together. Apply the mixture on your lips; you can do this one or two times a week. Beetroot has the pigments betanin and vulgaxanthin that brighten pigmented lips, while pomegranate is an antioxidant for preventing discolouration, and ghee has healthy fats for healing and moisturizing the lips.

TO GO THE CHEMICAL WAY OR NOT?

Natural DIY skincare can be your 'only' skin routine if you already have genetically healthy skin. But as we discussed in the chapter on skin, we are not the 'giraffes' of skin. We don't have perfect or 'normal' skin, certainly not all the time. Even with great genes, all of us are susceptible to environmental factors, such as sun damage, pollution, dehydration and ageing. DIY or home-made skincare solutions cannot address these effectively. It is much worse if you have skin with issues, for example, if you have acne-prone or sensitive skin or pigmentation. Home-made solutions do not work in such cases, and if you leave things unattended for too long, you can end up with a lot of scars and marks, which are much harder to get rid of.

WHY CAN'T ONLY HOME REMEDIES DO THE JOB?

- The percentage of actives is too low to achieve a measurable result.

- Many home remedies are irritating and can cause rashes (eg: lemon, the worst home remedy ever! Causes sun allergies, burns, irritation).

- You may be allergic to a home remedy.

- Too much scrubbing will remove the epidermis and damage your skin, so home scrubs with besan or ubtan are too irritating.

- For proper results, TRUST SCIENCE. It uses nature as its basis and makes it more efficacious.

Case in point: A client comes in with a dark depressed patch on her forehead that's visible from a distance.

Client: 'Doc, I don't know how this happened!'

Dr K: 'What home remedies are you using?'

Client: 'I used some lemon juice on my skin, before going out on a day picnic!'

Dr K (screaming inside): 'WHAT!'

Lemon is a known photosensitizer, which means it makes you really sensitive to the sun. So when you go in the sun after even brief exposure to lemon on your skin, you get rashes that look dark, red, depressed or swollen, and they are not pretty. And that glow you think you are getting from lemon? It's the same as doing an off-the-shelf chemical peel with an ingredient that is halfway effective but with too many side effects.

What's the benefit of science? If I am going to give you a chemical peel, I will choose ingredients for your skin type, for your lifestyle and ones that work with minimal side effects. Our 'chemicals' are based on years of research and we know how to use them.

Another case in point:

Client: 'I have too many painful zits on my face but I only use natural home remedies! How can this be?"

Dr K: 'Which home remedy have you used recently?'

Client: 'Oh! The cinnamon face-pack was wonderful! I read on the internet that it's great for acne-prone skin.'

Dr K (seething with anger, shaking fist in the air): 'WHYYY?'

Cinnamon is a well-known irritant and can trigger rosacea. Rosacea can often show up as painful pimples. The truth is that you can't fully diagnose your skin on your own, and experimenting without knowledge can cause serious damage.

CHEMICALS ARE NOT EVIL

- It's a myth that all things chemical are bad. All nature is chemical.
- We can't live without chemicals.
- PLEASE don't use the word 'chemical' and decide all chemicals are evil. Because then, you wouldn't exist. Join me in worshipping at the altar of chemicals. Okay, you don't have to worship them. But what you must know is that when you look for a solution, you should not be looking for 'natural' or 'chemical'. You should be looking for safety. And both natural or chemical things have specific safety profiles. You just have to know what they are. The danger of using only natural, because you think it's safe, is that you ignore the risks and end up with side-effects without any results.
- Water is a chemical. You, as a human, are made up of chemicals. Nature is a compendium of chemicals. Natural things such as snake venom are counteracted by medical lab-made anti-venom. Everything has its place and everything has its risk. Too much water is also toxic, did you know? Balance your fear with knowledge.

Sure, allopathic science has its limitations and its side effects. But we know what they are, and we also know their benefits. And all your home remedies are essentially using the base of all those active ingredients in top products out there.

Another self-remedy most people are guilty of is taking supplements without caution. Many supplements, especially when taken without proper knowledge, have lots of side effects. Vitamins can have adverse effects on your body, and can even cause diseases if overdosed. Do you know vitamin B12 can cause zits? Just because it seems 'healthy and natural' doesn't mean it's side-effect-free. In the same way, homoeopathic and ayurvedic medications also have side effects, even though they are essentially 'natural'!

Everything you do has a side effect. Just know what you are doing and navigate through it. When you need results, please go to a specialist to avoid serious side effects.

A DIFFERENT WORLD

The other, most important, truth is that we inhabit a world very different from the one our grandmothers, or even our mothers, lived in. The pollution in our environment is at its worst. It can cause acne, photo-ageing, pigmentation and more. The blue light from our screens and devices is problematic, causing early ageing, sagging, pigmentation and a host of other problems. The ozone layer has weakened over the years, and therefore, the UV rays are stronger. About 70 per cent of skin ageing is caused by the sun. We have a lot more HEV light exposure from our phones, which causes the same side effects as those caused by UVA rays. We have been exposed to many of these problems since a very young age. What you are exposed to when you are younger affects how you look when you are older. It is cumulative skin damage.

Stress-Mess

Let's not forget the most significant factor: stress! Look at how we live our lives today – the goals and expectations we have from ourselves, the balance of work and personal life, managing social media and presences, the expectation to be better parents, the struggle to live a better life. We are busier than ever. And while we are more mentally active, we are less physically active. Physical activity greatly contributes to a healthier lifestyle and healthier skin. People in the older generations were less anxious. Today, we are more connected, but it has also made us more anxious. We constantly want to know what the world is up to. Stress shows up on your skin big time. It shows up as pimples, as PCOS, as pigmentation.

Also, the food that we eat now is less healthy. There are more antibiotics and hormones in our food. It is not 'natural'. There are pollutants in our food and water, and they impact us in various ways. So, our lives today are a lot more adulterated than they were for our predecessor generations. All of this triggers inflammation in the system, which then worsens how our skin looks or responds.

It is important to know that your skin is your envelope. It is not designed to be perfect. It is designed to protect and express what is going on inside your body. Your skin is your signal mechanism. It signals that there is a problem. It is your guardian angel. And traditionally, your guardian angel is not supposed to be beautiful. It's not a part of its duty. But we expect it to be. Now, in addition to performing its duties, our skin also has to look good. We want our guardian angel to be perfect and beautiful and clear and supple and dewy and glowing. Phew!

The lens of love

When it comes to solutions that have been passed through generations in our homes, we attach a certain reverence and tradition with them. If our grandma recommended something for our skin, we accept it with love and use it because of love. But if you look at your grandma, even with great skin, she looks like a grandma. Through our lens of love, she looks beautiful and we want to hold on to that feeling of beauty. But in terms of skincare, when we look beyond the lens of love, we can see that sometimes our skin is not the same as that of our grandmothers. What we want from our skin – for it to look young, supple and radiant – may not necessarily be the same objective that our grandmother has for her skin. Our grandmother wants to maintain her skin as she ages. So, for our individual skin goals, we need to look beyond the lens of love, accept the reality of our skin, and look at skincare objectively.

DR K'S PRO-TIP

Home-made solutions and grandmother recipes for our skin, however, do teach us one thing that I too deeply believe in. That is, to not over-manipulate your skin. I don't believe in over-prescribing products or treatments. I want your skin to be healthy and as naturally maintained as possible. This is why I make you practise skin fasting and ensure that you also examine your diet and have a wholesome approach towards the maintenance of your skin.

What is a skin fast?

In my prescribed skincare routine, Sunday is skin-fasting day, wherin you only cleanse, moisturize and sunblock, possibly with as few products as possible (cleansing can even be done with just water). Or you can do a mask every Sunday, without any actives in your skincare regime that day.

You are an individual

You must understand that you are an individual! What works for someone else, may not work for you. Your skin is your own. It will react differently from others. You are a unique genetic code. No one on this earth has ever been like you or will ever be like you. So, why expect your skin to behave like everyone else's? It's not going to. My mantra is: love and accept the uniqueness that is you. Embrace it. And look at your skin from that perspective.

If you want to try home remedies or DIY solutions or stay 'natural' – by all means, do. But be objective about it. Be open-minded about the fact that it may or may not work. Give yourself a deadline. If you are trying a home remedy for acne, and it does not improve in one month, or three or even six months, then maybe it is time to treat it medically. I can understand that we all feel more comfortable with certain solutions. If you feel more comfortable with a home remedy, try it out. If it works, great. If not, be open to the idea of a different solution. Listen to your skin.

Don't hold on to traditions or family remedies just because they have worked for others in the family. Your skin is very important. If it is causing you suffering, don't continue to suffer. Get it the help it needs. There are treatments available for everything. Acne, pigmentation, scars, ageing – all are treatable or manageable. You can take an approach that works best for you. Try an integrative approach, which is my approach. You can do it holistically, or whatever is comfortable for you. But we should never ignore an entire science because we are scared.

At the end of the day, everything chemical is natural and everything natural is chemical.

7 CLEAN BEAUTY MYTHS!

1. Clean beauty should be preservative-free

All beauty products that last longer than three days must have a preservative in order to avoid bacterial or fungal contamination.

It's impossible for a skincare product to exist without preservation. Now, because people are concerned about parabens, we have a slew of other preservatives that are used. They may sound better, but typically, they are less studied than parabens are. So, just because it may be paraben-free, it doesn't mean it's preservative free. And you don't want a preservative-free skincare product, because it will give you a skin infection or affect the stability of the product!

2. Parabens are EVIL[13]

Traditionally, parabens were used as a preservative. Methylparaben, ethylparaben, propylparaben, butylparaben and isobutylparaben are all types of parabens that have been around since the 1950s, and have been used to prevent bacteria and fungus from growing in skincare products. All skincare products typically need some form of preservation. Did you know that 90 per cent of grocery food items have parabens in them? They are that ubiquitous – you just can't escape them!

Now, there is some data that has shown intact parabens in breast cancer cells in one small study with twenty people. It is possible that cumulative exposure to parabens could be an issue, and hey, even the EU has banned parabens. But, in the USA, parabens still exist because science is yet to establish a causal link between cancer and endocrine disruption and parabens, especially since the quantities used are very little, 0.1–0.3 per cent. Further, other preservatives are less studied and may even be more irritating than parabens. So, if you are getting an amazing skincare product that has a little paraben in it, don't freak out. You can balance it out with an overall paraben-limited regimen knowing that the jury is still out on parabens, and there is no reason to get worried given it's pretty much everywhere.

3. SLS must be avoided

What is SLS? SLS is sodium lauryl sulphate – a type of surfactant or detergent that cleanses and lathers. It's present in most shampoos and cleansing products because it's highly effective at cleansing and foaming. Let's be clear, SLS is a known irritant – if you apply it on dry eczematous skin, or if you put it on your skin and cover it up with a patch and leave it on for forty-eight hours. But are we doing that with our shampoos on a daily basis? NO! SLS is a perfectly acceptable ingredient for normal use if you need some foam and want to feel clean. Avoid it if you have dry skin or dry scalp or hair, or if you tend towards eczema or psoriasis or other skin conditions where the barrier is in disrepair. Simple! In the pursuit to avoid SLS, people end up using SLES, another type of detergent, or other different versions of surfactants, simply because they are scared of SLS. But are they getting any value from it? No.

You just want a gentler cleansing agent with less foam to prevent dryness. That's about it. The hype about SLS is a waste of time.

4. Clean beauty is chemical-free

I've said this before and I will say this again. Everything is a chemical, including water. I hate when people say 'chemicals are bad'. We are all one big chemical, guys; without chemicals, we would be dead.

5. Only use toxin-free products

This terminology is simply infuriating, and incorrect. Did you know that if you drink too much water, it can be toxic? What is the definition of a toxin? Any ingredient that is used at a proportion greater than the recommended dosage can affect the body negatively and be considered a toxin. No product can accurately be called toxin-free. It's bad marketing; don't fall for it. You are all better than that!

6. Vegan- and cruelty-free beauty is clean beauty

Even if a product is vegan, it can still contain parabens, SLS, silicones, you name it. Vegan simply means that no ingredient is derived from animals; it doesn't mean that the skincare is 'clean'. So, a 'clean beauty' product can have animal-derived collagen in it, while a vegan product can have propylene glycol. Further, 'cruelty-free' means that the product or its ingredients weren't tested on animals for efficacy. That's it. Any ingredient can be in it as long as it wasn't tested on animals; it has no bearing on safety for humans.

7. Clean beauty is the only kind of beauty products to use

Clean beauty is an artificial term designed to sell a subsect of skincare products. What exactly is clean, clearly no one really knows. In my book, a clean regimen simply means avoiding artificial fragrances and colours, because they are more likely to cause allergic reactions, as well as parabens as much as you can, because the data is up for grabs. Other than that, use everything in moderation and based on your skin type and comfort. Then look for efficacy – the mirror will thank you, and you will stop falling for marketing hype that doesn't serve you.

5

LISTENING TO THE SONG OF OUR BODIES
LIFESTYLE DISORDERS AND DISEASES

Client: Dr K, what is wrong with my hormones?!

POLYCYSTIC OVARY SYNDROME (PCOS)

PCOS, or polycystic ovary syndrome, now affects nearly 30 per cent of adult women and has become an epidemic of truly epic proportions. Every other woman who comes into my clinic has some symptom or aspect of PCOS, and I know it can really be troublesome. And since I am here to ensure you glow inside out, let's talk about PCOS. Then, I will talk about two other common diseases, thyroid and diabetes, and how they affect your skin and hair too!

'Syndrome', not 'disease'

Since it's so insidious and prevalent, we now consider PCOS to be a syndrome more than a disease. What does that mean? It means that you are not diseased – it's not an illness that can be cured. Your body has metabolically changed, so that it is now much more sensitive to things it could handle before with ease. And your body is showing you that by being more acne-prone, having more hair growth on the face, experiencing hair fall from your scalp, excess weight gain, period irregularities (although not always), insulin sensitivity, and more. To have PCOS means that your body has become a highly trigger-sensitive machine – that your body is triggered by changes in food, weather, moods, stress, schedule changes, jetlag, etc. I understand it sounds upsetting. So, what do you do now? Now, you have to actually LISTEN to your body. You have to care for your body. You have to love your body, and accept it. You are now FORCED to own it and step up to the plate.

That means: eating healthy, exercising, stress management, skincare, haircare. Regular CARE! Can you do this? Yes, you can. And if you do, your life will change. For the best.

Now, let's get down to the hairy details.

When I see a patient with acne as an adult or extra hair anywhere on their body or face, or if they seem to have difficulty in getting rid of their facial hair no matter how many laser hair removal sessions they undergo, I have to first rule out PCOS. Yes, I know that sounds crazy, because there was once a time when you had to first wait and see because PCOS was rather rare. Now, it's so common, we just assume it! After all, as an adult, why should you have zits? Why should you have hair growing out of your chin? In most cases, it is not normal, and the magic of your body is telling you, 'Babe, it's time to make a change!'

Decades of stress, eating high glycaemic, sugary, high carbohydrate, processed foods, avoiding vegetables in our diets, frying a lot, and allowing our phones and screens to determine our schedule – has now shown up on and in our bodies. Our skin is screaming, our body is crying, and our hair is shedding. This is PCOS.

SIGNS OF PCOS

You can have one or some or all of these symptoms; everyone reacts differently:

- Acne on your jawline or chin

- Resistant or recurrent acne

- Hairy beard-like growth on your face

- Excess hair on your chest, tummy, back or thighs

- Hair thinning and hair fall from your scalp (yes, it really sucks that you get more hair on your face and body, and less on your head ... the worst.)

- Irregular periods (although many people with PCOS have regular periods)

- Weight gain or difficulty losing weight

- Insulin resistance or early pre-diabetes

- Acanthosis nigricans (darkening on neck, underarms, knuckles – a sign of insulin resistance)

- Difficulty with fertility

- Ultrasound with multiple cysts

MYTHS

'My period is regular so I can't have PCOS'
FALSE
PCOS can show up as other symptoms while your periods can come like clockwork.

'Only women can have PCOS'
Both TRUE and FALSE

In the form that it comes to female bodies, yes, only women experience it but there is something similar in men, where they experience early balding and insulin resistance.[14]

'My hormones are normal, so I can't have PCOS'
FALSE
You just need the symptoms above to have PCOS, even if blood tests, ultrasound and periods are normal.

'PCOS is curable'
FALSE
It's a lifestyle condition and needs permanent and regular monitoring.

'PCOS means you will never have kids'
COMPLETELY FALSE!
It's simply your body telling you that you need to take care of yourself, which you will and you can. Some women may struggle with fertility but many will not. And usually, it's manageable, so do not fret.

It's not all bad news! Everyone responds differently but for most:

- The acne will go. It may recur, but we can do preventative care to manage it.
- The facial hair will go away with the right laser hair removal; this is manageable.
- The body hair will also go away with laser hair removal!
- The hair fall can stop.
- The weight gain can go away.
- The insulin resistance can be reversed.
- You can have babies.

Breathe, you got this!

A few tweaks, a few changes, and life goes on beautifully. In fact, it becomes better, healthier and you feel more 'lit' than you have ever been.[15]

PMS ACNE or premenstrual acne is the acne you get a week before your period starts, or even around your ovulation time – and this is not PCOS!

What is it? This is where either you have excess estrogen, or you have relative estrogen dominance, meaning even if your estrogen levels are normal, they are in the wrong proportion relative to the progesterone levels.

Who gets it? Nearly anyone can get this, but in my practice, I tend to see it more in populations above the age of thirty. It is a travesty for us womankind!

DR K'S PRO-TIP

How to treat it? Magnesium is a great supplement for this – 300–350 mg taken at night for three to six months has been shown to improve PMS acne and symptoms significantly. Also, taking 40–100 mg of vitamin B6 has been shown to be beneficial, but don't take exceed the dosage.[16]

Spot Treatment?

For tiny pimples: Try a salicylic-acid-based spot treatment. Brands such as Clearasil, Neutrogena, and Clean & Clear have 2 per cent spot treatment products that costs almost nothing; they are great for tiny whiteheads and pustules.

For big bumps: My favourite mix is a combo of Vaseline and Mario Badescu's drying lotion, which is elemental sulphur (no, it is not sulpha; sulpha is a chemical compound that is a component of some antibiotics, while sulphur is a natural element present in the environment and in our body). First put the drying lotion and then apply vaseline on top.

How can PCOS be managed?

First, we need to determine the type of PCOS – which we do with blood tests, symptoms and ultrasound. I also check for estrogen dominance, which shows up as those zits and PMS symptoms you get around your period or around ovulation. This is not PCOS: this is a relative excess of estrogen to progesterone.

I also insist on a few changes:

- **Diet** – To be discussed more in the following chapter. But cut out high glycaemic foods (meaning foods that raise your blood sugar levels really high, such as white sugar, maida, potatoes and chips), to help reduce insulin resistance. Increase the fibre content in your diet. Avoid dairy as it has lots of hormones in it and is hormonogenic, and can worsen the imbalance in your body. Intermittent fasting is a great addition as well.

- **Exercise** – Exercise forty-five to sixty minutes a day, five to six days a week. This helps reduce stress, which can otherwise worsen your PCOS, and will also improve insulin resistance.

- **Stress reduction** – Understanding yourself, keeping anxiety and obsessive thoughts at bay, practising meditation – all this will help reduce the amount of cortisol in your body and manage the symptoms of PCOS.

- **Sleep** – Reduce screen usage, and follow your circadian rhythms. Sleep on time by 10 p.m., and wake up on time. I know it sounds crazy, but your body will thank you. Screens are stimulatory, so you won't be able to sleep if there's too much screen usage at bedtime. Stop work at a decent hour. Find a way to relax your mind and sleep for at least seven to eight hours.

- **Hydrate hydrate hydrate** – This is obvious. Don't make me write the word 'hydrate' again. You are made of water. Drink water.

- **Supplements** – Based on the type of PCOS you have.

My medication mantra

I try to treat PCOS mostly without oral contraceptives or hormones, because coming off the pill has its own trauma, and the pill just seems to hide the issue, not cure it. We saw this with diabetes as well. We started medicating diabetes, instead of lifestyle modification, and now we have learned how reversible diabetes can be, especially in the first year. If we can change the lifestyle, we can avoid a lot of medications. Food is the real medicine. Of course, food and diet can't cure everything, and you may need medication, but let's use it only when absolutely needed. You have the power to change your life. Only you can! LET'S EMPOWER OURSELVES!

Besides diet and lifestyle changes, I often recommend a slew of supplements and work with you to see what will help and won't. Remember, supplements are effective and can create positive changes in your body. But they can also have side effects, just like medicines can. So, we watch and change and remove as needed.

For those who want to get rid of excess facial hair, we do a custom LHR protocol to give results. I am sure you can find a credible clinic or specialist near you for laser treatment. Don't expect miracles, but work with your aesthetic specialist or skin doctor, and talk about your needs and issues. Trust me, communication is everything.

Now, here is some detailed information on everything you need to know about PCOS.

PCOS or Polycystic Ovary Syndrome

PCOS is basically androgen excess (high male hormones) in the body or a specific hormonal imbalance. This is a hormonal disorder common among women of reproductive age. Women with PCOS may experience infrequent or prolonged menstrual periods or excess male hormone (androgen) levels. They may also have normal periods and standard hormone levels, but exhibit symptoms that are consonant with PCOS. Yes, PCOS can be very insidious.[17] 'The Endocrine Society advises clinicians to diagnose PCOS using the 2003 Rotterdam criteria, although recommendations differ across guidelines. According to the Rotterdam criteria, diagnosis requires the presence of at least two of the following three findings: hyperandrogenism, ovulatory dysfunction, and polycystic ovaries.'[18]

Symptoms of high androgenism

- High androgens (testosterone, Dihydrotestosterone, 17-hydroxyprogesterone, DHEA-S, Andronostenedione) in your blood
- LH/FSH ratio greater than 2:1

- Insulin resistance (can show up as elevated fasting or postprandial [post-meal] glucose or insulin, or as elevated HBA1C)

- Facial hair or excessive hair on the body in specific areas in women (hirsutism)

- Alopecia, i.e., hair loss or thinning on the scalp

- Recurrent acne or acne in adulthood

Ovulatory dysfunction

- Oligomenorrhea or irregular periods

Polycystic ovaries

- Presence of multiple cysts on ovaries, as shown in pelvic ultrasounds

Hirsutism

What is hirsutism? It's basically a male pattern of hair growth seen in women. It's usually defined on the face but can also show up on the body. Hirsutism is the scientific term for the presence of coarse hair in females in male-like distribution, that is, on the back, face, chest, neck, stomach and some more unlikely places. This happens in females when the androgen levels are high, which means there is more than the usual amount of testosterone being produced.

Here is a diagram of all the different areas that excess hair can show up on the body and face, and how to grade the growth.

All that upper lip and beard hair is not just your parents' genes! Unfortunately, hormones are to blame too.

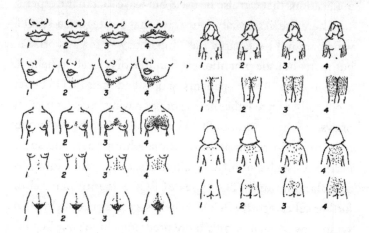

Hirsutism can be a part of PCOS, or it can simply be your genes. About 10 per cent of the time, we can't find a hormonal cause of hirsutism, but we believe that is because there is a peripheral conversion that happens in the tissues themselves, making them more sensitive to male hormones, which cannot be measured by modern science. Hirsutism is treatable, and modern laser hair removal is a god-sent boon for those of us cursed with excess hair.

Now, a few more details on PCOS in a nutshell, starting with the different types of PCOS that are there. I will discuss the types of PCOS below, along with the natural remedies for each type. For medicated treatment, typically, oral contraceptives with an anti-androgen effect are preferred, or anti-androgens such as aldactone can also be given, while metformin is also used to help with insulin resistance, which will also help reduce the male hormones in the body. There are a host of other medications that can also be used, but leave that to the experts.

There are essentially four ways that I categorize PCOS, which are not necessarily the allopathic way to categorize it, but many holistic practitioners find this organization helpful, and I find that it helps patients understand their PCOS better too. In addition to either having or not having irregular periods or cysts in the ovaries, all PCOS is characterized by symptoms of hormonal irregularity, excess male hormones, and some insulin resistance or high insulin levels, along with a low level of inflammation.[19] The types of PCOS mentioned below further subcategorize PCOS to help segregate people by what symptoms are significantly more predominant in your PCOS.

1. **Insulin-resistant PCOS:** If your insulin levels are high, then your insulin is driving your androgens and you have insulin resistance and insulin-resistance PCOS. Here, I look at whether your post-prandial (two hours after a meal with 75 gm of carbs) insulin or glucose is elevated in contrast to your fasting insulin or glucose. The beginning of insulin resistance usually shows up in your post-prandial results – because you begin to make more insulin than you needed to before for the same amount of glucose in your blood, meaning that your sugar is 'resistant' to the same amount of insulin, thereby requiring more insulin to keep your blood sugar stable. The problem is that insulin stimulates and downregulates other hormones in the body, leading to acne, and even increases in male hormones later on, resulting in hair fall and more.

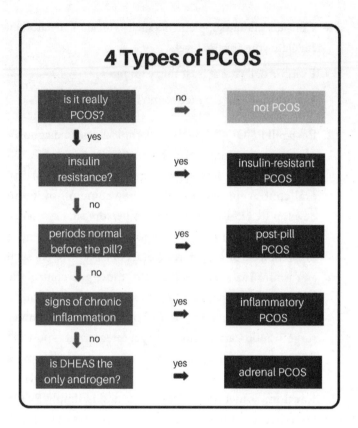

4 Types of PCOS

is it really PCOS? → no → not PCOS

↓ yes

insulin resistance? → yes → insulin-resistant PCOS

↓ no

periods normal before the pill? → yes → post-pill PCOS

↓ no

signs of chronic inflammation → yes → inflammatory PCOS

↓ no

is DHEAS the only androgen? → yes → adrenal PCOS

Treatment

- Go for a low-carb and high-protein diet, exercise more, and reduce your stress to fix your insulin levels. You want to avoid high glycemic foods, or foods that stimulate insulin levels too high, and you really want to change your lifestyle. Stress will aggravate all conditions, so rest, healthy sleeping and eating patterns, and exercise and meditation are key!

- Consider adding supplements such as inositol, to naturally regulate your insulin levels.

- Exercise daily for at least thirty minutes

- Medications such as metformin may be needed.

2. **Post-pill PCOS:** While this is technically not a diagnosis, it's a great way to categorize a temporary form of PCOS when someone has regular periods before starting oral contraceptives, and then they come off of it and develop PCOS-like symptoms. A person can experience a temporary surge in androgens when coming off a drospirenone or cyproterone oral contraceptive pill such as Yasmin, Yaz or Diane. Basically, those pills control the high male hormones in the body, so once you are off them, you can get a spike in them afterwards. This temporary surge in androgens is enough to get categorized as post-pill PCOS. Usually, this condition is temporary and resolves over six to twelve months as your hormones rebalance.

   Caution: Sometimes, it continues and is simply PCOS them because the OCP (oral contraceptive) was likely treating an actual problem, but once you are off the medicine, the problem is no longer being treated. In that case, other treatment may be required. Then you are not Post-Pill PCOS! Post-Pill PCOS is specifically for those who had normal periods before going on the pill and no signs of insulin resistance, and only have a temporary rise in male hormones after coming off the pill.

Treatment

- Diet is key! You want to reduce any foods that may exacerbate the androgens in your system, including dairy, whey or casein protein powders or high glycemic foods.

- Take natural anti-androgen supplements if needed for three to six months under the guidance of your doctor. These include fenugreek supplements and rarely saw palmetto – but these should be discussed with your doctor first.

- Be patient! Typically this is temporary and not real PCOS.

3. **Inflammatory PCOS:** Chronic inflammation can stimulate the ovaries to make too much testosterone, which can trigger PCOS. I consider this inflammation to be stress: if you have chronic stress, that will translate into inflammation, which can eventually lead to PCOS. Here, the concept of inflammation is highlighting that many of us just keep surviving each trauma and each difficulty without giving ourselves the rest and care that we need. Ultimately, denying your own stress and ignoring it will show up in the body. Moreover, recurrent illnesses, poor eating habits, poor lifestyle contribute to inflammation in the system, which can exacerbate a predominantly inflammatory driven type of PCOS. Symptoms of inflammation may be unexplained fatigue, IBS (irritable bowel syndrome), headache, joint pain, eczema, rosacea, psoriasis, hives and many other symptoms.

Treatment

- Identify the cause of inflammation and treat that. This means, look back: have you been eating unhealthily? Drinking too much? Not sleeping well? Do you have a lot of anxiety? Have you had recent health scares or personal traumas and losses, during which you did not care for yourself well? Do you sacrifice your well-being for your work or for your family? Inflammation or stress isn't just illness; it's also emotional. Don't ignore your own needs.

- Avoid inflammatory foods and include anti-inflammatory foods in the diet. (The food chapter will give you more details)

- Work on your gut with probiotics, prebiotics and avoiding common triggers (see next chapter).

- Treat any food sensitivity and histamine intolerance.

- Anti-inflammatory supplements can be helpful, but diet and lifestyle will be the most effective in helping you deal with this.

4. **Adrenal PCOS:** PCOS is characterized usually by insulin resistance and high levels of male hormones. The majority of the time, those male hormones originate from the ovaries, but in 20–30 per cent of cases, those male hormones, particularly the hormones DHEA-S and 11β-hydroxyandrostenedione, come from the adrenal

glands that sit on top of the kidneys.[20] This is because the ovaries and adrenals affect each other, and also because insulin resistance and high insulin levels common in PCOS can trigger the adrenals.[21]

Treatment

- Reduce stress and practise meditation. Stress is a trigger for the adrenals, so reducing it will benefit you.

- Eat a low glycemic diet. Since high insulin levels can trigger the adrenals to make DHEA-S, reducing the amount of insulin you make by eating foods that trigger insulin less, will make a difference.

- Avoid artificial sweeteners, because they often create the same insulin response as sugar!

- Eat happy foods, i.e., foods such as nuts, seeds, fruits, dark chocolate, which release happy chemicals. Also include green leafy veggies.

Your doctor can diagnose the type of PCOS you might have, and you can get treatment, along with a wellness and diet plan designed specifically for your needs.

～

Here are some general guidelines that you can follow regardless of the kind of PCOS you have. This is kind of a 'best-practice' guide for any type of PCOS. Starting with the most important: foods that you need to avoid.

Foods to avoid if you have PCOS (and if you're acne-prone)

PCOS and acne can be treated in a similar way when it comes to diet, as both tend to be caused by hormones.

- **High Glycaemic Index Foods:** Avoid white bread, sugar, flour, bananas, grapes, raisins, mashed potatoes, rice cakes, muffins, cakes, cookies and soda.

- **Dairy:** Milk leads to a rise in testosterone levels as it contains a protein that limits normal testosterone processing in the body. With the body unable to manage testosterone naturally, the levels just keep rising. As testosterone levels tend to rise in PCOS, dairy makes the problem worse.

- **Caffeine, Alcohol and Beverage:** Drinks with refined sugar, such as colas, soda, sweetened juices and syrups, are a complete no for women with PCOS. Alcoholic drinks have a far greater physical impact on a woman's body: they can lead to sugar overload, insulin resistance and affect fertility.

- **Gluten:** Cutting down on gluten or following a gluten-free diet will reduce inflammation in the body. Go for more gluten-free meals, which include poached eggs, quinoa, soups, salads and green vegetables.

- **Sugar:** Quick fact, when I was nineteen, I stopped consuming sugar and sugar substitutes entirely. I also quit caffeine and turned into an angry monster, but that's another story. My taste buds got used to not having sugar, and even now, I find most things to be too sweet. I believe it helped make me healthier in the long run.

For those of you who cannot go cold turkey, I hear you – try taking my dark chocolate from me, you will have to pry it from my cold dead fingers. Solution? Cut your sugar intake by half every month. Whatever you do, do half of it and, then slowly, half it over the next few months, and you will end up with the same effect.

With PCOS, you are much more likely to be sensitive to sugar, and then subsequently end up with insulin resistance and diabetes. The signs of this insulin resistance can show up on your skin, as dark patches on your underarms, groin, knuckles, neck and knees. These are called acanthosis nigricans. Insulin resistance itself is problematic because it increases your likelihood of getting heart disease, organ damage, nerve disease and more. And from a purely physical point of view, insulin resistance will age you faster, give you pigmentation, make your skin thicker and drier, and overall, significantly more damaged. It damages your collagen too, so all that sugar in your bloodstream is not only damaging your organs, it's also preventing you from looking and feeling your best. If you must have sugar, you can have a little jaggery, or even coconut sugar, but try to go cold turkey and remove sugar from your diet entirely.

Now that we have discussed all that you *cannot* (or should not) eat, let's talk briefly about all that you can eat to help with your PCOS:

(TAKE A SCREENSHOT!)

FOODS THAT HELP IN PCOS (AND WITH ACNE):

- **Vegetables:** Eat four to six servings of vegetables every day, such as kale; spinach and other dark, leafy greens; broccoli and cauliflower. Healthy fibre-rich foods such as legumes and vegetables provide necessary nutrients for the body.

- **Fruits:** Eat only one to two servings per day. For fruits with a high concentration of sugar, such as mangoes, cherries and oranges, one serving is enough. For those with a lower concentration of sugar or a lower glycaemic index, such as papaya and grapefruit, you can have two servings. Dark red fruits, such as red grapes, blueberries, blackberries, and cherries are excellent.

- **Protein:** Include protein with every meal because proteins have a stabilizing effect on the sugar that is released by carbohydrates. Fatty fish, including salmon, tuna, sardines, and mackerel are good. Eggs, chicken, and nuts, such as pine nuts, walnuts, almonds, and pistachios, are also good sources of protein. Dals or lentils and beans are all great sources of protein. Remember to soak your nuts and beans/legumes overnight to remove phytates (phytates from the skins of these nuts can make your stomach uncomfortable and result in bloating).

- **Fats:** Eat 2 to 3 servings of fatty fish every week in order to load up on essential fatty acids that are beneficial for controlling PCOS symptoms. If you are vegetarian, snack on healthy nuts and seeds, such as almonds, walnuts, pecans, sunflower seeds and flax seeds, that are rich in monounsaturated and polyunsaturated fats. Healthful fats, such as ghee, olive or coconut oil, as well as avocados and coconuts, can be added to the diet too.

Some key food rules:

- KEEP IT WHOLE: Consume whole grains instead of processed and refined foods, and whole fruits instead of fruit juices in order to maintain optimum blood glucose and insulin levels.

- EAT A LOT MORE FIBRE: Eating foods rich in fibre leads to a slower, consistent and controlled rise in blood sugar and insulin levels. The more fibre you eat, the healthier your gut will be!

The crucial thing to understand is that PCOS is a lifestyle disease, and we need to alter our 'lifestyle' to deal with it entirely. Food and diet are one part of it. Besides those, we need to also take care of our emotional and physical wellbeing, starting with reducing stress.

Ways to combat PCOS

Stress management

Stress is a huge part of our lives. If left unchecked, it transforms into a lifestyle disease and becomes a major cause of PCOS.

Stress reduction is crucial when managing PCOS. So, what do we do with all this stress we are under?

Let's go to the root of it. What exactly causes stress? We are consistently in contact with the world, constantly receiving messages, DMs, emails and notifications. This constant updating is stressing us out. In the olden times, people used to write letters, which would take two to three weeks to reach a person! People would wait to hear from their loved ones and would have time to think and respond. When there were fights, one would send a letter to a trusted elder, and he would respond and then plan to visit months later. Everyone would be forced to manage themselves better. Nothing was immediate with timestamps and double ticks. Now we live in times where we want our every emotion to be resolved in a minute. We are bombarded by news every second, by WhatsApp messages every nanosecond, social media updates, video calls, emails – my god, the list goes on! There is no personal space or time to self-soothe anymore.

Also, we want everything, all the time: social media, and media in general, has made it seem as though we all need to be perfect with perfectly curated homes, gorgeous dressing styles, with great careers, amazing social lives and a mantra of impeccable wellbeing. The explosion of external demands on what we must be is taxing. Sleep and circadian rhythms have been sacrificed at the altar of Netflix and social media browsing, all of which have altered our brain. This is in addition to the contaminated foods that we consume (more on this in the next chapter). Further, pollution is a major stress on our system, and we can barely take out time or consideration for self-care, health and sleep. No wonder we are one big ball of stress.

Now, how do we deal with all this stress?

Here's what I do:

- Mornings are crucial: I do ten minutes of meditation or at least a motivational 'rampage' in the mornings. It helps me set my mind positively for the day. I think about what I am grateful for and connect to that. I also take this time to focus on the goals for the day.

- I avoid scrolling social media too much in the morning because it genuinely makes me feel sensitive and a little hopeless without any reason. Everyone has the right to do what they want, and no one is as happy as they present themselves on social media. Despite knowing that, I get emotional, and I can't imagine what the average teenager may feel like.

- Turn off your device post 8 p.m. You will thank me. Your neck will have fewer lines (no more tech neck!) and your double chin will improve from all that time not spent bending over a cellphone. Your mind will be able to concentrate and you'll sleep better.

Physical Exercise[22, 23]

Physical movement[24] and exercise[25] are crucial in managing PCOS.[26] PCOS has an associated risk of type-2 diabetes and cardiovascular disease. Studies have shown that physical exercise can reduce this risk significantly. So, get up and move it!

If you don't usually exercise, I would recommend going for a walk or run at least, whichever works for you. Walks are calming and centring. It's your chance to move your body and not be on your phone (I would seriously advise only using your phone to listen to music, if at all). Forty-five minutes or an hour of brisk walking is excellent cardio and will get your heart pumping in a happy way. But if outdoors or walking or running is not your thing, you can always do yoga, pilates, weight training, Barre and so many other things. Post COVID, many studios and gyms offer home classes too, if you want to exercise in the comfort and safety of your house.

Our lives in the digital age are essentially sedentary, so anything that gets you moving is good for your PCOS and is good for you.

Mindfulness

Beyond stress management and physical exercise, it's important to look at what triggers PCOS-like symptoms at a deeper level, and that's when we focus our attention on our thoughts. Our thoughts trigger our emotions and constant stressful thinking can show up as various physiological manifestations in our body, including hormonal imbalances and PCOS. So, what do we do with these thoughts?

Write them down. Sometimes your thoughts are all over the place and might just be pointless: maybe your friends are not talking about you, or you feel in a funk because you lost your keys one day, get anxious thoughts about the world ending (trust me, it isn't).

I am not asking you to dismiss your thoughts. Acknowledge them, no matter how negative or silly they may seem. Write them out. When we see our thoughts on paper, we can see them for what they are and can calm down the emotions that they are triggering.

The idea is to learn how to regulate our emotions. Sometimes, for deeper unresolved trauma or complicated thoughts, it is crucial to seek out therapy and learn a way to manage them.

Surround yourself with real, authentic positivity (beware of toxic positivity and toxic people). Read, watch, listen to self-empowering authors. Some of my favourites are Abraham Hicks, Joe Dispenza, Eckhart Tolle, Michael Singer, among others. You can start with them or find your own favourite TED talks, podcasts, YouTube channels, books (reading is a great stressbuster if you are into it, and it also takes away from screen time). Figure out your formula for being mindful and stress-free. Because you deserve it more than you know.

THYROID

Other than PCOS, there are two major culprits that commonly affect our skin: thyroid and diabetes. Both manifest in different ways, and if you find any symptoms of these, you should make that trip to the doctor soon.

Approximately one in 300 people have hypothyroidism, and the number one cause of it is autoimmune. Women get it more frequently than men do, and the likelihood increases as you get older. Other causes, such as a simple viral illness or post-pregnancy thyroiditis (inflammation of the thyroid), can also be a trigger, as can iodine deficiency, or a thyroid tumor.[27] But the most important thing to know is that, usually, thyroid disease is not preventable.

Now, if you have hypothyroidism or subclinical hypothyroidism, where your TSH is normal but there are antibodies circulating against your thyroid, your skin and hair will show some signs. These include, but are not limited to, the following:

- Dry and coarse skin
- Cold extremities
- Sparse and brittle hair
- Hair fall
- Hair loss on the outer third of the eyebrows
- Brittle or ridged nails
- Puffiness, swelling or water retention
- Depression

It takes at least three to six months to normalize these symptoms once the thyroid begins to get treated.

Often, I will also prescribe a diet to reduce inflammation in the system and see if the issues resulting from thyroid resolve faster, but typically the thyroid does require treatment. And no, your thyroid doesn't get addicted to the medication.

There is also something called hyperthyroidism, where you make too much thyroid hormone. Here you will find symptoms like:

- Moist skin
- Excess Sweating
- Weight loss
- Hair fall
- Swelling on the shins (pretibial myxedema)
- Protruding eyes
- Itching
- Nail changes
- and more!

This requires medical treatment immediately. So, please see your doctor ASAP if you see these symptoms!

DIABETES

Diabetes is when either your body doesn't make enough insulin or your body can't use the insulin the way it should. This results in an overload of sugar in the bloodstream, which causes downstream effects on organs such as the skin, heart and kidneys.[28]

Visible signs of diabetes on the skin include:

- Necrobiosis lipoidica, which are patches of swollen and hard skin that begin as bumps. Digital sclerosis is hard, waxy and thickened skin that looks like an orange peel and occurs particularly around the fingers and toes, spreading through the forearms to the back, shoulders or chest. These can even occur on the legs and feel tight and heavy. Sometimes, you can't even straighten your legs due to it.

- Recurrent blisters
- Recurrent skin infections
- Open sores known as diabetic ulcers
- Diabetic dermopathy or shin spots

Diabetes is very toxic to the skin: the excess sugar will circulate and damage the collagen in the skin, resulting in thickened and damaged skin. Diabetes can also lead to a host of skin diseases that can be hard to treat. That's why your lifestyle and what you eat become so important in managing the disease.[29]

While diabetes has severe outcomes on these end-organs, even pre-diabetes can show up on your skin.

One example is acanthosis nigricans. It is a fancy word for dark skin on the back of the neck, under arms, groin and knuckles. These are clear signs that you will either get diabetes or you are well on your way there. When you see acanthosis nigricans on someone's skin, you know the first thing to do is diet and lifestyle intervention; skincare comes after that. The skin gets thick and dark in those particular areas, and sometimes even in other areas, so it needs to be treated internally too, not just externally.

Read the next chapter to learn more about how to heal your body with what you eat.

6

WE ARE WHAT WE EAT

'The ham's on your pillow,
The egg's in your sheet,
The bran muffin's rollin',
Down under your feet,
There's milk in the mattress,
And juice on the spread-
Well, you said that you wanted
Your breakfast in bed.'

– 'Sorry I Spilled It' by Shel Silverstein

It's true! We *are* what we eat. And we need to know what we are eating. I am sure you have seen older relatives with clear acne-free skin their whole lives, while your entire generation may be plagued with zits. And this world has a literal epidemic (a bad word in our time) of PCOS. Our grandparents have always insisted on drinking milk to make us strong, and now doctors are telling you that dairy is bad. You keep eating your vegetables but, for some reason, the pores won't go. Everyone keeps talking about gut health, but your gut just doesn't listen. How many berries must you eat before you glow like a fresh-looking peach? 'Oh, just drink more water and your skin will be perfect!' 'Keep dairy at bay, to keep those zits away!' All these dilemmas to sift through before you end up having a mental breakdown and tearing at the little hair left on your thinning crown.

Don't worry, we are going to break it down. We are going to talk about why your food isn't doing you good and how to make it work for you, why your water is a problem and what to do about it. And in the end, I'll provide you with a guide – that I also give to my patients – on what to eat for your particular skin and hair needs.

First, our food is not what it used to be some decades ago. Our water is full of toxins, our food genetically modified (GM) and heavy on pesticides, insecticides and fertilizers. Did you know it's been proven that an apple now has 60 per cent less nutrition than it did in the 1950s?[30]

Add to that, what we are choosing to eat is also a problem. Sodas, packed juices, MSG, corn starch, refined flour, sugar, more sugar, preservatives, artificial colours and flavours – the list goes on! And the marketing machines of big foods haven't helped. Why are grains and dairy still such a big part of our food pyramid, when tonnes of data shows that they are not great for us? Why were we told to follow a high-carb, low-fat diet for so many years, even though with this diet, our population gained weight, diabetes became more rampant, and cardiovascular disease became increasingly common? And we ended up with things such as trans fat, which jam our arteries.

We desperately need to talk about what we eat and drink, because what goes inside you, shows outside, especially on your skin (and more).

WHAT IS WRONG WITH THE WATER WE DRINK?[31]

It is no secret that our bodies are about 60 per cent water and we cannot survive without it. So, the kind of water we drink is extremely important for our survival. Lead, arsenic, mercury, copper and radioactive compounds, such as radium, can leak into our water, putting us and our children at risk for cancers, brain damage, reproductive complications and more.[32] Our skin, too, witnesses the effect with rashes, pigmentation and more. Other toxic ingredients that we are exposed to include perfluorooctanoic acid (PFOA), which is from Teflon coatings and can cause kidney issues, problems with menopause and other adverse health effects. Perchlorates, nitrates, chlorine are some other offenders as well. Pesticides, herbicides,[33] endocrine disruptors, such as bisphenols, also populate our water supply. The list is endless, and this might also be a factor in the rise in PCOS, resulting in that acne and hair fall we so desperately hate. In the past fifty years, our water has become increasingly hazardous, and it is affecting us and our children in many subtle ways that we will only be able to understand generations from now.

So how do we ensure our water is safe? Certainly do not drink tap water unless it has gone through the proper process of filtrations.

DR K'S PRO-TIP
Drink water that has been boiled or treated by reverse osmosis, distillation, or filtration with an absolute 1 micron (or smaller) filter.[34]

To remove 97–99 per cent of pesticides, endocrine disruptors and heavy metals, you need to use reverse osmosis or solid block carbon filters. Look for filtration systems with at least two to three stages and ultrafine tiny filters for best results.

Now, the next crucial question is about how much water to drink. Are those 'hydrate, hydrate, hydrate' calls for real? Does drinking a lot of water keep us healthier? What is the correct amount of water to drink?

Water helps us excrete toxins, regulate our temperature, help blood flow, among many other functions. If it's 60 per cent of our body, it is integral in every single way. Even your skin will look worse without enough water – rough, dull, enlarged or more visible pores, fine lines, under-eye wrinkling, the list goes on. On the other hand, if you drink too much water, you can actually end up with water toxicity! (And the number of times you end up going to the bathroom will also feel pretty toxic).

The right amount of water drink is about 2.7 litres for women and 3.7 litres for men in a day. If you sweat a lot, are exercising, drink alcohol or coffee and tea, then increase the intake by one glass of water for each activity. Water that has electrolytes in it hydrates the best. Coconut water in the summer is wonderful and also helps prevent acne due to its mineral content. And there is a reason why people in India love nimbu soda: it's got salt or sugar, or both, are electrolytes that help keep you hydrated. I believe that sprinkling black salt on our fruits/vegetables in India has been a way of staying hydrated in the hot weather, since fruits and vegetables have lots of water, while the salt adds the electrolytes!

WHAT'S WRONG WITH THE FOOD WE EAT?

Those of us lucky enough to get trustworthy organic fruits, veggies and meat are the rare few. (Studies have shown that even organic food can be contaminated, and that false marketing campaigns claiming organic produce are rampant). In his landmark study, University of Texas researcher Donald Davis and his team found that there have been 'reliable declines' in the amounts of 'protein, calcium, phosphorus, iron, riboflavin (vitamin B2) and vitamin C'[35] in the food we consume. According to Davis and his team, the reason for this is the change in 'agricultural practices' to produce crops that are better in 'size, growth rate, pest resistance', while ignoring nutrition. It's all about capitalism! So, even when you are eating all the right things, they just aren't working!

How many clients have told me something on these lines: 'But I eat so well, yet my skin is bad.' Well, you are eating all those amazing oranges, but they have 60 per cent less vitamin C. There is a reason why we are all stuck on supplements these days. (Please don't take this to mean you should eat fewer fruits and vegetables. Food sources of vitamins are always better than supplements, so keep eating your veggies and fruits religiously.)

The other issue across the spectrum is the proliferation of processed food. As our lives get busier and time is always short, a lot of people have turned to the most easily available solution: processed foods, which is actually the worst option!

Processed foods, being convenient to consume, have taken over our lives. Eating foods that are far removed from their origin and are made in factories, not in nature, cannot be good for us. Examples of this: processed juice, pop-tarts, 'fruit-flavoured' cereals. What does that even mean? It means that it's an artificial chemical, which tastes like fruit, that's been added (while you've been made to believe that it is more 'natural'). Processed foods are nothing but high-glycaemic foods, with lots of sugar, refined flour and a lot of chemicals. All those foods that claim to be healthy but aren't include boxed juices, cereals, 'whole wheat atta' (typically, chock full of refined flour with very little actual wheat), and more. Also, kids' snacks are the worst culprits: the claims of being packed with extra vitamins or being full of fruits and vegetable benefits are far from true. Typically, they are just easy for kids to eat, while adults feel like they are helping their children with nutritious alternatives, when in fact they are just being duped by marketing. You know why this is? Because these packaged foods (no matter how carefully you pick them) are full of sugar, refined flour and/or have a high glycaemic index, meaning they cause a rapid spike in insulin once consumed. These types of foods can not only increase your risk of getting diabetes, heart disease, strokes (all of which cause mortality as noted above), but they can also affect your gut health, make your digestion poorer, and give you dementia.

But let's focus on the relationship between food and skin now. What can food do to your skin? The worst culprit of all is sugar. Excess sugar can give you acne, severe acne, as it increases sebum or oil secretion. Teenagers will get acne easily, and adults will have drier and more damaged skin. It can also increase hair fall. In fact, early-onset male pattern balding is associated with insulin resistance. We talked about this in the chapter on hair, but I am reminding you because it's important. It's considered a kind of male 'PCOS', although without the ovaries. So, you can imagine how much it can increase the risk of PCOS for the women out there.

We are getting pigmentation on our necks, underarms, knuckles and groin due to insulin sensitivity (called acanthosis nigricans) because of all the sugar we are eating. We are experiencing fat deposition around our waists as well, and the cellulite is worsening. Our skin is ageing way faster, and that dewy glow looks further and further away from us as we consume this junk more and more.

HERE IS A SUGAR HIT LIST

- Acne
- Hair issues
- Balding
- PCOS
- Ageing
- Dry and itchy skin
- Skin tags
- Thick and hard skin
- Blisters
- Skin ulcers
- Acanthosis nigricans (darkening of the neck, knuckles, underarms, groin)
- Rare skin diseases
- Increased skin infections, among many other issues you already know about[36]

It must sound weird, right? How does a bit of quick sugar age you, make you look older? All that sugar accumulates and lives in your bloodstream. It's not supposed to be there, but with the modern lifestyle and eating habits we have, there is a lot more just hanging around.

And you know what it does: it creates AGEs, or advanced glycation end products. These little chemicals made from excess sugar accelerate ageing and chronic disease. The same glycation increases the signs of ageing and makes skin thicker and discoloured. AGEs get attached to collagen, elastin and fibronectin – the most important components of skin structure responsible for elasticity, suppleness and firmness. They damage these proteins and also make them resistant to removal, so new collagen cannot be then formed, thus ageing the skin rapidly.[37] They also makes the skin more rigid and more resistant to repair. Now this is common knowledge, but AGEs affect nearly every other cell in the skin as well. They affect keratinocytes, making them renew slower, with poorer balancing of the skin. They target the immune cells, increasing inflammation. They target fibroblasts, thereby reducing suppleness, tightness and skin renewal.[38] So, I'd think twice before opening that snack packet or carbonated drink.

Artificial sweeteners are not the solution either, by the way. Aspartame has been shown to have neurotoxic side effects and is associated with Parkinson's disease and even fibromyalgia. Moreover, artificial sweeteners often cause the same insulin response as sugar, so you aren't preventing diabetes in any way through them.

I have had patients reduce their sugar intake and see drastic improvement in their health – the kilos melt off, their pigmentation reduces, acne gets better and they look younger by years. I've had even ten-year-olds limit their sugar, and their health and skin became so much better. Cutting sugar can even prevent the early onset of acne in pre-teens and teens. By pampering them with unhealthy high-sugar snacks, you are only hurting them in the long run. You can save on the money you spend on junk food while also giving yourself and your kids the gift of a healthy body and skin.

~

Next stop, dairy. When I tell my clients to cut out dairy, they look at me like I have grown horns on my head. 'But I need milk to grow strong! Where will I get my calcium from? What about my bone strength?' they ask incredulously. I look at them with a deadpan face and tell them that data from Scandinavia shows that excess intake of milk actually increases fracture risk, and you can get calcium easily and in a better way from non-dairy sources.[39] Sadly, few believe me.

Did you know?

In a study in California, it was found, and I quote: '47,355 adult women were asked to recall what they ate during their high school years. Only cow's milk was found to be linked to acne. Women who drank 2 or more glasses of skim milk a day were 44% more likely to have acne than others.'[40]

So many clients have seen enormous changes in their acne and even PCOS by cutting out dairy or cow's milk. Don't stress: you can still eat yoghurt or curd. Why is this? Yoghurt and curd are fermented, and it is believed that fermented dairy has less inflammatory lactose and galactose, while having anti-inflammatory and gut-boosting probiotics, thereby mitigating a lot of the side effects of unfermented dairy.[41] Probiotics also reduce the secretion of IGF-1, which is a known trigger of acne.[42] Regular milk has whey and casein in it, which stimulate hormones such as IGF-1, which then affect our hormones further, often resulting in zits. Further, from an anecdotal point of view, I believe the milk is adulterated with antibiotics, and fertilizers and pesticides, which have unknown effects on our bodies. And even if the milk is organic, the cow's own hormones will still be a part of the milk you drink. We have enough hormones already and don't need to be adding a cow's hormones in the mix.

Now, how do you replace it? Well, I love almond or coconut milk – even rice or oat milk is acceptable – and you can make these easily at home, too. For those who must have cow's milk, although I don't prefer it, you can drink limited amounts of A2 milk, which is actually the milk that is endemic in Indian cows, buffalos, camels and goats. It lacks a type of casein that is present in A1 milk, and is thus easier to digest and slightly less inflammatory. Please note it's still cow's milk and can still cause acne. And lactose-free milk as a replacement of dairy, you ask? Lactose-free milk is still dairy, its just without a particular sugar called lactose. It's the same milk, it still has whey and casein, it still has every other ingredient, just without the lactose. It can still cause acne. IT'S STILL DAIRY.

PS: When we talk dairy, we primarily mean milk. Cheese and yoghurt, in limited amounts, are still allowed. So please don't freak out, no one is banning your dahi!

ALMOND MILK[43]

Ingredients:

Almonds, 1 cup

Water, 4 cups

Method:

1. Boil the water. Add the rinsed almonds.
2. Cover and let them soak for thirty to forty-five minutes.
3. Once the almonds are soaked well, drain the water and peel the almonds.
4. Blend the peeled almonds with water in a blender. Once blended well into a paste, strain once or twice.
5. Collect the almond milk in a bottle or jar and store it in the fridge.
6. Fresh almond milk stays good for three to four days.

Notes:

The almonds can be soaked overnight too. Don't throw away the leftover almond paste. Use it to make cakes, cookies or bread.

OAT MILK[44]

Ingredients

Steel-cut or rolled oats, 1 cup

Water, 4 cups

Unrefined salt, ¼ tsp.

Cinnamon powder, ⅛ tsp. (optional)

Method

1. Soak the oats in drinking water for at least two hours. Drain and rinse the oats. Set aside.

2. Add the oats to a blender with one cup of water. Blend until you obtain a smooth paste; this will take three to five minutes.

3. Add the rest of the water, salt and cinnamon powder. Blend well.

4. Store in a glass bottle for no more than a few days.

Notes

This recipe yields one litre of oat milk. If you are gluten-sensitive, you can use gluten-free oats. Skip the cinnamon if you have sensitive or rosacea-prone skin.

COCONUT MILK[45]

Ingredients

Grated fresh coconut or unsweetened shredded coconut, 2 ½ cups

Water, at room temperature, 3-4 cups

Method

1. Put the grated coconut in a blender with water, and blend on high till the coconut is ground well.

2. Strain the paste in a cheesecloth, muslin or fine sieve, and collect the first extract in a bowl or pan: this is the thick coconut milk or the first extract.

3. Put the extract back into the blender.

4. Add 1 to 1.5 cups of water, and blend again.

5. Strain and collect this coconut milk in another bowl and set aside. This is the thin coconut milk or the second extract.

6. Put back the coconut gratings in the blender. Add 1 to 1.5 cups of water and blend again. This is the thinnest coconut milk or the third extract.

7. Strain for the third time and collect the third coconut milk in the bowl in which the second thin coconut milk is extracted. You can also keep the third extract separate.

8. Your coconut milk is ready. Use it fresh in your cooking, or refrigerate and use later.

Note
If using unsweetened shredded coconut, soak the coconut in warm water for a few hours before blending.

~

Now, let's talk gluten! I believe gluten should be removed from the diets of those who are intolerant to it, or have a sensitivity to it (say you feel lethargic or heavy, or your stomach feels uncomfortable after consuming gluten-rich foods). If you have an autoimmune issue, gluten can trigger it even more. I have seen that removing gluten benefits people with psoriasis or eczema, but other than that, unless you feel uncomfortable or are genuinely allergic, there is no need to avoid it. Enjoy your gluten; just keep it at a low-glycaemic index. Avoiding high-glycaemic ingredients means keeping off foods that raise your blood sugar real fast, so maida is a definite no-no. Your skin will thank you, your zits will be under control, and you will save money on that concealer.

That gut feeling

The most important organ, when it comes to food intake, is the gut. Our gut does much more than just digest the food and extract the goodies from it: it also forms a protective barrier between our insides and the external world. So, keeping it healthy is super important!

A healthy gut feels good, and when your digestion is good, you get good absorption of vitamins and minerals from your food and inflammation is low. Now, what is a leaky gut? This is where the barrier is weak or 'leaky'. When your intestines allow stuff to pass through the intestinal barrier into the bloodstream, as opposed to outside through the natural process of going to the bathroom, you end up with a lot more immune system reactivity, because they see stuff that shouldn't belong and go on the attack! Unsurprisingly, the symptoms of a leaky gut can show up anywhere – from the gut to the joints, the skin, and the brain. It can give you rosacea, pesky zits, abdominal pain, bloating, headaches, and can be accompanied by diarrhoea, indigestion and/or gas. Fatigue, brain fog, confusion may also occur, and eventually, it may also result in nutritional issues, autoimmune diseases, inflammatory bowel disease or depression.[46]

I also believe that gut health is associated with how much weight we gain, so those who want to stay within a healthy weight limit may want to pay extra attention to the gut.

There are many reasons behind a damaged or problematic gut. Here are the six most likely causes of gut damage, leading to leakiness and inflammation:

1. **Pharmaceutical drugs**: Around two-thirds of NSAID (nonsteroidal anti-inflammatory drug) users have a leaky gut. Antibiotics also can clean out the good bacteria, leaving the bad bacteria to create those holes in the intestinal barrier.

2. **Stress and anxiety**: Stress and anxiety can cause a leaky gut, and a leaky gut can cause stress and anxiety: it's a vicious cycle.

3. **Dysbiosis**: The imbalance between the good and bad bacteria (and other microorganisms) that live in the gut is never good. Dysbiosis can cause symptoms such as bloating, cramping, brain fog, depression and many common intestinal maladies.

4. **Diet**: The dietary factor most likely to increase the leakiness of your gut is the intake of foods and drinks such as alcohol, sugar, refined carbohydrates and refined cooking oils. Vegetable oils made from corn, soya and sunflower are especially culpable. They are high in omega-6 and fatty acids, which are notorious for their pro-inflammatory effects.

5. **Smoking**: It's the habit that keeps on taking. It's also free-radical hell.

6. **Allergens**: Foods to which you are allergic or intolerant also create irritation and inflammation in the gut. It is important to notice how you react to every food that is on your table.

Any of these reasons (or many or all of them) could be causing us gut-trouble. So how do we fix it?

Here is your 'let's heal the gut' action plan. Take a screenshot, print it and pin it on your fridge to remind yourself how to take care of your gut.

1. **Take probiotics**: Start taking probiotic supplements containing friendly bacteriam which produce anti-inflammatory chemicals that fight the unfriendly ones and help protect the stomach environment.

2. **Eliminate sugar and refined carbohydrates**: Sugary foods and drinks trigger the release of large amounts of the hormone insulin, which in turn is a trigger for inflammation. The more insulin there is, the more inflammation there will be.

3. **Reduce vegetable oils**: Vegetable oils that contain inflammatory omega-6 are ubiquitous in ready-made meals and take-outs. To avoid the toxicity of these oils, it might be easier to cook all your food from scratch using butter, ghee or coconut oil.

4. **Avoid alcohol**: Alcohol is a well-known depressant, gut irritant, and a contributor to leaky gut syndrome.

5. **Increase vegetables in your diet**: Add as many vegetables as you can manage, especially the brightly coloured ones, including peppers, tomatoes, red onions and eggplants. Make sure that you also eat at least one portion each day of dark leafy greens, such as cabbage, broccoli and spinach.

6. **Include fermented foods**: Foods such as live yoghurt, kefir, sauerkraut and pickled vegetables increase the levels of lactic acid bacteria such as *Lactobacillus acidophilus*, which help in settling your stomach.

7. **Eat oily fish**: Omega-3 fatty acids, found abundantly in oily fish, are an important indicator of the gut-mind connection. Patients with depression have been found to have lower blood omega-3 levels than others.

8. **Review your medications**: Determine if you are taking NSAIDs (non-steroidal anti-inflammatory drugs) with your doctor and see if any alternatives are available. Also, ask your doctor when you can avoid taking antibiotics.

9. **Avoid allergens**: Gluten, which has a long association with leaky gut, is found in wheat, barley, rye and oats. If you suspect a leaky gut, avoid gluten.[47]

Food for Skin

Do specific skin concerns require eating or quitting certain foods? Can I improve my skin problems by changing my diet? Let's talk about your skin and food in deeper detail!

BASIC DIETARY GUIDELINES

Foods to limit (to once a week) or avoid completely

- Sugar
- Wheat
- Dairy (no paneer/milk/curd)
- Refined vegetable oils
- Bread and processed foods (once a week)
- Spicy foods
- Whey protein powder
- Too much caffeine (limit to 1-2 cups/day)
- Alcohol

Foods to consume

- Green leafy vegetables such as spinach and kale and highly pigmented fresh fruits such as blueberries and raspberries (no fruit juice)
- Protein (eggs, fish, nuts, seeds, lentils, chickpea/ kidney beans)
- Nuts (almonds/walnuts/cashews/pistachios/brazil nuts), a handful a day
- Seeds (chia/flax/quinoa/sesame/pumpkin/melon/ hemp/sunflower), 2 tbsp. a day

- Fish (omega-3-rich fatty fish), either salmon or small fish
- Whole grains (quinoa/besan/bajra/jowar/makka/kuttu/singhara)
- Red rice/kerala rice/matta rice/quinoa
- Healthful oils (ghee/coconut/mustard)
- Dark chocolates (above 75 per cent), 1 cube a day

Alternatives

- Whey Protein → Substitute with vegan protein powder (plant-based protein powder, peas, hemp and rice are typical substitutes)
- Sugar → Organic honey/dates/prunes/coconut sugar
- Dairy → Almond milk, coconut milk, oat milk (gluten-free), nut cheeses
- Wheat → Almond flour/coconut flour (for cookies/pancake/cheela), jowar (sorghum), ragi (millet)

Health Tips

Do:

- Chew each bite thirty times for proper digestion, because your mouth has digestive enzymes and it's biologically designed to carry out the majority of digestion. The stomach comes second, and the intestines are for vitamin absorption. If you do not chew properly, nutrients will not get absorbed well. Also, eat without distractions.

- Vegetables and fruits should be organic and GMO-free. All hormone-injected foods should be avoided.

- Exercise every day for thirty minutes and keep yourself hydrated all the time.

- Intermittent fasting (14-16 hours): You can have black coffee or green tea during the fasting period. Do it 1-2 times a week.

Don't:

- Use plastics and plastic bottles.

- Eat raw foods, such as salads, sprouts and fruits, after 4 p.m. Try not to eat solid food after 7 p.m. (clear broth/ vegetable soup allowed).

Now, let's get more specific. Maybe you want to work on your diet with something specific as the end goal. Maybe you want to look younger, or brighter, or just want to do something more nourishing for your sensitive rosacea-prone skin. Look no further, I break down the tips I give my clients on their specific skin concerns, right here for you.

ANTI-AGEING DIET

Ageing is the most common concern that no one – and I mean, no one – is a stranger to. Skincare is often designed around 'anti-ageing' which can sound rather unbelievable. Because, let's face it: we all have to age. Ageing is change. And we all change, every year, every decade. But does ageing have to mean bad skin? Not if I can help it. And not if you can help it.

Sometimes, a lot of what ages us, somewhat prematurely, besides genes, are environmental factors and a bad diet. Let's look at the causes of skin ageing. Free radicals, which are by-products of the metabolism process and environmental factors, cause ageing to a great extent.

What are free radicals? Formed by pollution, inflammation, smoking, metabolism and UV light, these are molecules that lack an electron, so they go around to perfectly healthy and happy cells trying to steal their peace and stability by trying to grab one of their electrons. They are like trolls on social media – just can't leave you alone in peace! Antioxidants are the defenders against these free radicals.

1. **Diets** comprising **high fat, processed food or fast food, fried food, packaged food, irradiated food, junk food margarine** and **starchy vegetables** create oxidative stress, resulting in the production of more free radicals.

2. **Alcohol** suppresses the formation of antioxidants.

3. **Polluted air,** especially in the big cities and towns, also creates more free radicals.

4. Drinking tap **water containing chlorine, fluorine and other harmful chemicals** and toxins produces more free radicals in the body.

5. **Lifestyle**-related problems cause the production of lesser antioxidants and more free radicals.

6. **Diseases** such as asthma, high blood cholesterol, cardiovascular disease, high blood pressure, diabetes, Parkinson's disease, and cancer fuels free-radical production.

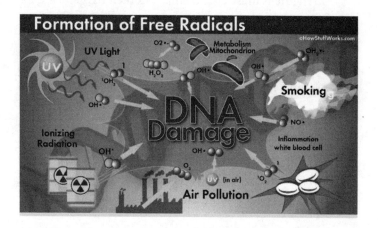

Most of these causes, especially the environmental ones, are unavoidable (and for that, I suggest you find a good skin doctor and work out a skin rejuvenation plan that works for you) but diet and lifestyle are things you can control, right? So, let's do it. Here are some points that you need to print out, cut out, memorize, tape to your mirror and read daily!

- Cut down alcohol and stop smoking! Those pesky wrinkles around your eyes and mouth, and early sagging and pores? Hello, cigarettes! That dull grey colour and pigmentation on your face? Smoking will do that. You know better.

- Get beauty sleep to rejuvenate your skin. Six to eight hours of sleep. Do it. If you feel rested, you will make better eating decisions too.

- Yoga improves blood circulation and concentration, strengthens muscles and enhances their oxygen-carrying capacity, keeps our body and fit by burning fat and helping it lose weight, thus slowing down ageing.

- Drink plenty of water as it hydrates your body and is essential for anti-ageing nutrients.

- Use HEPA air filters in your house.

- A balanced diet is of utmost importance to maintain healthy skin. Eat lots of fruits and vegetables that are rich in minerals and vitamins known for their anti-ageing benefits: check out the list below.

Superfoods for anti-ageing[48]

Foods that are antioxidant powerhouses[49]

BEANS

- Small red beans (dried) are the highest source of antioxidants in the world. In fact, it has been found that three out of five of the highest antioxidant potential foods are beans. Beans fight free radicals and are extremely beneficial for healthy ageing.[50]

- Red kidney beans have plenty of antioxidants and overcome free radicals easily.

POWER-PACKED VEGETABLES

- Kale is full of antioxidants and slows down the reaction of free radicals in the body and is thus good for your skin.

- Green leafy vegetables such as broccoli, cabbage, and cauliflower are not only beneficial for the prevention of cancer and heart disease, but they also impart a bright and youthful glow to the skin.

- Spinach contains lutein that helps improve vision clarity.

- Carrots are full of antioxidants and vitamin A.

- Russet potatoes are a good source of antioxidants and have anti-ageing properties.

COLOURFUL FRUITS

- Tomatoes contain antioxidants and lycopene. The latter prevents cancer (prostate cancer), muscular degeneration and has anti-ageing properties.

- Berries (blueberries, raspberries, strawberries and blackberries) are abundant in fibre, vitamins, minerals, antioxidants – all these help in the prevention of cancer and heart disease, and check age-related damage.

- Red grapes have resveratrol and quercetin that strengthen heart function. The antioxidants act as free-radical scavengers and help keep blood vessels unblocked. Resveratrol also protects from gastric problems, stroke and arthritis.

- Pomegranates, known to contain beneficial nutrients and antioxidants, help reduce blood pressure and the impact of cardiovascular and heart disease.

TEAS AND SPICES

- Ground cloves, cinnamon and oregano have a rich content of antioxidants.

- Green tea prevents degenerative diseases and reduces the likelihood of cancer, heart disease and stroke.

> DR K'S PRO-TIP
>
> Antioxidants are a great add-on for anti-pigmentation benefits as well!

VITAMIN C

- Vitamin C helps facilitate youthful skin and collagen synthesis. Natural sources of vitamin C are citrus fruits, such as oranges and lemons, and also in some vegetables.

VITAMIN A

- Vitamin A protects the body from solar radiation severity. Sources of vitamin A are carrots, broccoli, kale, tomatoes, etc.

Vitamin E

- Vitamin E helps keep the skin healthy and youthful. It fights skin ageing from within. Sources of vitamin E are sunflower oil, grains, oats, nuts and avocado.

Roots

- Ginger assists the digestive system, eases arthritis and reduces free radicals in the body.

- Radish and turnip are known to be excellent anti-ageing foods.

- Garlic is packed with antioxidants and is known for its anti-ageing benefits. It fights free radicals and prevents blood clotting.

Nuts

- Remember, peanuts are not nuts; they are legumes! And they are well-known to be inflammatory, so don't add those to your anti-ageing diet.

- Walnuts are good for anti-ageing as they are abundant in omega-3 fatty acids.

- Nuts strengthen the immune system and remove dryness from the skin. Avoid rancid nuts as they are abundant in free radicals.

- Pecans act against degeneration, fight free radicals and are beneficial for anti-ageing.

DR K'S PRO-TIP

Soak the nuts and peel them to avoid putting stress on your digestion. The phytates in nut skin can cause cramping and discomfort, so soaking and removing the skin makes them much more palatable to the gut.

HEALTHY FATS

- Flaxseeds and avocados are chock full of omega-3 fatty acids, which are anti-inflammatory and heart-healthy.

- Avocado reduces cholesterol levels in the body, helps maintain healthy skin due to its vitamin E content, and reduces the signs of ageing.

YOUR ANTI-AGEING MEAL PLAN

First thing in the morning	1 glass detox juice (amla, lemon, ginger, cucumber, holy basil [tulsi], mint, turmeric, black pepper). Mix these ingredients in a blender with a liquid base of coconut or mineral water.
Breakfast (pick one not all)	1 cup oatmeal (use gluten-free oats, almond or coconut milk, 1 tsp. organic honey and 3-4 strawberries, 2 tbsp. pomegranate)

	2 small walnut protein pancakes (2 tbsp. gluten-free oats, ½ cup coconut flour, 2 tbsp. chopped walnuts, ½ tsp. baking powder, 1 tbsp. vanilla extract, 2 egg whites, ½ cup almond/coconut milk) Use olive oil for making pancakes. **1 cup gluten-free oats namkeen dalia** (add green beans, carrots, tomato) + **half a mosambi (sweet lime)** **Strawberry and kiwi smoothie** (½ apple, ½ banana, ½ kiwi, 4 strawberries and 1 tsp. honey) **with egg white spinach omelette**
Lunch (pick one not all)	**1 bowl red rice pulao** (1 cup boiled red rice + lots of green veggies according to taste) + **1 plate green salad** (fresh cucumber, cherry tomatoes, kale, celery, lettuce, sprinkle juice of half a lemon) **Apricot and almond quinoa pulao** (1 cup cooked quinoa with 4-5 apricots and almonds cooked in olive oil with green and black olives) + **1 plate green salad** (fresh cucumber, cherry tomatoes, kale, celery, lettuce, juice of half a lemon)
	1 cup mix veg (cabbage, peas, carrot and beans) + **1-2 quinoa roti** (stuffed with 2 tbsp. gluten-free oats) + **1 plate green salad** (fresh cucumber, cherry tomatoes, kale, celery, lettuce, juice of half a lemon) **1 cup red/brown rice + 1 cup fish curry + masala bhindi** (3-4 pieces only) + **1 plate green salad** (fresh cucumber, cherry tomatoes, kale, celery, lettuce, juice of half a lemon)

	1 cup green/yellow pepper and peas veg + 1 makka/bajra/jowar roti (stuffed with 2 tbsp. gluten-free oat bran) + 1 plate green salad (fresh cucumber, cherry tomatoes, kale, celery, lettuce, juice of half a lemon)
	1 cup mushroom, peas, spinach and yellow pepper veg + 1 besan roti (stuffed with 2 tbsp gluten-free oats) + 1 plate roasted beet, plum and kale salad
	1 cup broccoli rice with 1 cup egg curry + 1 plate green salad (fresh cucumber, cherry tomatoes, kale, celery, lettuce, juice of half a lemon)
Evening snack (4-5 p.m.; pick one)	2 walnuts + 10 almonds + 1 cup cranberry juice
	3 tbsp. seed mixes + 1 cup strawberry juice
	1/4th avocado with 1 glass guava juice
	2 tbsp. pumpkin seeds + 1 glass blueberry juice
	1 small plate sweet potato chat + 1 cup grape juice
	4-5 apricots + 1 cup cranberry juice
Dinner (pick one)	100 g pan-fried salmon fish + 1 cup mixed vegetable home-made soup
	100 g lemon herb salmon + 1 cup home-made soup (put green veggies, rosemary, parsley)
	Sesame-soy salmon (fish) with carrots soybeans (put bedding of Bok choy or spinach) + 1 cup chicken soup
	Fish cutlets (use oat bran for binding) + 1 cup tomato soup

	2 cups grilled veg (any green vegetable; sometimes, you can have soya as well)
	100 g barbecued tofu (add green and red pepper, mushroom and some herbs in it) + 1 cup lentil soup
	100 g grilled spicy chicken with 1 cup vegetable soup
Night detox	1 glass detox water (add jeera, saunf, ajwain in water and boil it)

The IDEAL Plate[51]

- Five to seven servings of fruits and vegetables daily: 1 source each of vitamin A, vitamin C, vitamin E, and the rest in antioxidants

- 1 serving of nuts

- 1 serving of seeds

- Four to five servings of beans/lentils every week

- About 70–80 per cent of your food should be fruit, vegetables, nuts and seeds.[52]

According to the *American Journal of Lifestyle Medicine*, what we need is a 'nutritarian diet'. This is basically 'vegetable-based, utilized a wide assortment of colourful vegetables, root vegetables, green vegetables, peas, beans, mushrooms, onions, nuts, seeds, and some intact whole grains'.[53]

ROSACEA AND FOOD

We have already discussed the diet you need in order to treat acne and PCOS, and you can refer to chapter 4 for it. Coming to rosacea, it is a common complaint of many clients, and we have talked about it earlier in this book as well. It is also called 'sensitive skin' or 'blushing'. While it is often caused by external factors – such as exposure to sunlight, hot or cold temperatures, strong winds, hot baths, intense exercise, and stress – what you eat can also be a cause. So, here are some quick tips I give my clients for eating right to prevent rosacea.

Dietary guidelines for rosacea

There are many foods and drinks that trigger the inflammatory responses brought on by the condition, such as flare-ups, redness, dilated blood vessels, and thickening of skin.

Don't eat these:

- Vegetables such as tomatoes, hot peppers, carrots, beets, eggplant, onions, radish and spinach.

- Drinks such as alcohol and hot beverages, i.e., hot coffee or tea (which can dilate blood vessels and contribute to facial redness).

- Sugar and starchy foods such as artificial sweeteners, cookies, refined sugar, chocolate, candies, fruit juice, potatoes, breakfast cereals, barley, pasta, bread and white rice.

- Strong spices such as ginger, cumin, black pepper, fenugreek and cloves. Spices that contain capsaicin are triggers for rosacea (capsaicin is found in certain spices and peppers).

- Cinnamaldehyde-rich foods such as tomatoes, citrus, cinnamon and chocolate should be avoided. Foods containing cinnamaldehyde are triggers for rosacea. (I got a big zit from cinnamon because I have rosacea, so telling you this from personal experience, guys!)

- Dairy products, such as cow milk, curd, buttermilk, butter, cheese, cottage cheese and other dairy products, can often trigger rosacea.

- High-histamine foods, such as fermented alcoholic beverages (wine/champagne/beer), and fermented foods (sauerkraut, vinegar, soy sauce, kefir, yoghurt, kombucha). Vinegar-containing foods (pickles, mayonnaise, olives). Dried fruits and nuts (apricots, prunes, dales, figs, raisins, walnuts, cashews and peanuts).

- Nitrate-rich foods or preserved meats, such as bacon, salami, pepperoni, luncheon meals and hot dogs.

Eat these:

- Light vegetables such as asparagus, cucumber, sweet potatoes, leafy greens, pumpkins, broccoli, cauliflower, celery, okra, lettuce, green beans and zucchini.

- Soothing spices such as coriander, cardamom, saffron and fennel.

- Anti-inflammatory foods such as salmon, chia, flaxseeds, turmeric.

- Non-citrus fruits such as grapes, melons, mango, pear, watermelon and cantaloupe.

- Non-vegetarian foods such as salmon fish, turkey, chicken, poultry and eggs. (If you are a vegetarian, skip this one.)

- Low-histamine foods such as gluten-free grains, rice, quinoa, pure peanut butter, non-citrus fruits and leafy herbs (herbal tea).

- Cooking oils such as olive oil, coconut oil and ghee (ghee is Indian clarified butter that aids in proper immune system function).

- Dairy substitutes such as coconut milk, rice milk, hemp milk.

GLOW BONUS

Want a natural glow? Pre-teens, teenagers and adults tend to have a lack of antioxidants in their diet resulting in some skin dullness. They also tend to get tanned more easily because they don't have enough antioxidants in their skin and body to counteract oxidative damage from external elements, resulting in melanin secretion and deposition, which is a sign of damage to the skin. Apart from the antioxidant levels in the body, the gut also needs more nutrition, with prebiotics to curb inflammation. And then, finally, we get to nutritional boosting with vitamin C, vitamin A, iron, calcium, zinc, trace minerals and more.

I have an awesome recipe in the form of what I call the '7-Juice', which covers all the nutrients you need to really glow from the inside out. This is an all-in-one juice with the essentials to promote healthy skin and hair!

Ingredient	Nutritional benefit
1. SPINACH/KALE/ CELERY A healthy handful of spinach	Vitamin A, vitamin C, antioxidants and iron (for anti-ageing, rejuvenation and promotion of healthy hair)
2. SUPER-SEED MIX 1 tbsp. of chia + sesame + sunflower (and pumpkin seeds if you want) Keep this seed mixture pre-mixed in your pantry and add a couple tablespoons to your juice mix!	Fibre, omega-3 fatty acids, calcium, iron and zinc (for GI ease, glow, non-dairy calcium source, so you can avoid acne-causing dairy, healthy hair and acne prevention)
BEAUTIFUL BERRY MIX Blueberry + cranberry + 1 amla (a handful each of both berries) Add some goji berries or a teaspoon of acai powder for a superfood boost if you can source them.	Antioxidants and vitamin C (for anti-ageing and rejuvenation)
POMEGRANATE Seeds from half a pomegranate.	Antioxidants and punic acid (punic acid helps with inflammation in sensitive skin or inflammatory skin conditions, such as acne or rosacea)

Ingredient	Nutritional benefit
ANY IN-SEASON CITRUS The juice from half of a citrus fruit (my favourite is mosambi)	Vitamin C (for rejuvenation and radiance)
HONEY/DATES/PRUNES 1 tbsp. (or more to taste)/ 2 dates / 3-4 prunes	Iron, antioxidants, digestive ease, anti-bacterial properties (and to add sweetness) If this drink tastes sour or bitter, add honey/dates/ prunes, as per your taste.
UNRIPENED BANANA 1 whole banana	Prebiotic and digestive assistance (there is a theory called 'The Gut-Skin Axis', which shows that there is a proven, strong correlation between gastrointestinal health and skin health)

Method:

Mix all seven ingredients in a blender with a liquid base of your choice. I recommend coconut water for light days and almond/ coconut/oat milk when you want something a bit creamer.

If the drink is bitter and sour, add two dates instead of so much spinach, as it is rich in iron and will give you a good taste as well.

Drink every morning before food for best results.

ANTI-INFLAMMATORY DIET

Inflammation and food

If you have a skin conditions such as eczema or psoriasis or some form of autoimmune disorder, or if you have recently recovered from COVID or another illness, then you have a lot of inflammation in your system. All that inflammation will affect your organs, as well as your skin and hair. So, your goal is to reduce that inflammation the best way you can, and that is through your diet. Gluten, dairy, peanuts, omega-6 fatty acids, sugar, processed foods with high-glycaemic indexes, and trans-fats are all well-known to be inflammatory, and should be removed from your diet ASAP! If you reduce the inflammation in your body, a lot of your symptoms can also be reduced.

Foods to avoid

To determine what foods may be causing or worsening the inflammatory reaction, a person should go for an elimination diet. This diet involves avoiding some of the most common foods known to particularly cause eczema.

- Citrus fruits
- Dairy (30 per cent of kids will have an allergy to cow's milk)
- Eggs
- Gluten or wheat

- Soy
- Spices, such as vanilla, cloves and cinnamon
- Tomatoes
- Some types of nuts

People with dyshidrotic eczema, which typically affects the hands and feet, should avoid foods that are high in nickel.[54] These include:

- Beans
- Black tea
- Canned meats
- Chocolate
- Lentils
- Nuts
- Peas
- Seeds
- Shellfish
- Soybeans

Avoid the following foods, which can be harmful for people with eczema, who can also have oral allergy syndrome, i.e., sensitivity to birch pollen:

- Green apples/pears
- Carrot
- Celery
- Hazelnuts

Foods to eat

- Fish, a natural source of omega-3 fatty acids that can fight inflammation in the body. Types of fish high in omega-3s include salmon, albacore tuna, mackerel, sardines and herring.

- Foods high in probiotics, which contain bacteria that promote good gut health. Examples include yoghurt with live and active cultures, miso soup and tempeh. Other fermented foods and drinks, such as kefir, kombucha, and sauerkraut, also contain probiotics.

- Foods high in inflammation-fighting flavonoids. Examples of these include colourful fruits and vegetables, such as apples, broccoli, cherries, spinach and kale.

Let's talk about some fun food trends! Here are two that I absolutely love and see becoming popular in the near future!

TREND ALERT: IV NUTRITION BARS

IV drips are now here to stay. As medical residents, hungover or tired doctors would get a banana bag – or a drip with fluids and electrolytes – to feel rejuvenated and be able to work. The same thing can be given to people with jet lag and bad hangovers. Also, vitamin C IV has been shown to boost immunity and reduce the duration of colds and short viral illnesses, and was even studied for COVID care as well. Further, as we discussed earlier, even if we are eating correctly, our food is less nutritious than before. We absorb almost 100 per cent of what is in the drip, so what better way to replete your vitamins, minerals, antioxidants and fluids than with a quick IV shot? I believe, when done in moderation, these IV bars can be a value addition to your good health. But, be careful, don't do too many. If you have health issues related to kidney, liver, heart, sugar/insulin, and hypertension, ask your doctor if it's safe for you.

TREND ALERT: INTERMITTENT FASTING

Intermittent fasting is quickly growing as a trend among conscious eaters. It is pretty amazing, and it's great for your skin! Watch your acne improve, your PCOS get better and, as a bonus, weight loss too.

Intermittent fasting involves meal timing cycles and schedules that restrict energy. It is a voluntary and controlled fasting. During fasting, a person must not consume any food or calories – calorie-free drinks such as water, black coffee and tea are allowed.

Fasting longer periods can result in autophagy: this is the state the body reaches after fasting, which allows the body to remove dysfunctional cells and gives more health benefits.

Types of intermittent fasting

1. **Twice a week (5:2):** In this method, you do two days of fasting and eat a normal healthy and balanced diet on other days. On fasting days, calorie intake should be around 500 calories and you should also focus more on high-protein and high-fibre foods.

2. **Alternate day fasting:** This method involves fasting every other day. Limit your calories to 500 on fasting days and have a healthy and balanced diet on normal days.

3. **Time-restricted eating (16/8 or 14/10 method):** In this method, you have to set an eating window. Most people already fast while they sleep, so this method will be really convenient as you extend the overnight fast by skipping breakfast and not eating until lunch.

   There are two ways of doing this fasting:

i. 16/8 method: In this method, ensure a gap of sixteen hours in between the last meal of the day and first meal of the next day.

ii. 14/10 method: In this method, ensure a gap of fourteen hours in between the last meal of the day and first meal of the next day.

4. **The 24-hour fast:** This method involves fasting completely for a full day, for twenty-four hours. Fasting can be done from breakfast to breakfast or lunch to lunch and, on normal days, eat a healthy and balanced diet.

Health benefits

1. Intermittent fasting helps in **weight loss.** The eating cycle allows people to control their appetite, eat less each day and track their eating habits better. Fasting can increase metabolism by up to 4 per cent, which helps burn calories quicker. It also increases your energy levels.

2. Intermittent fasting has **anti-inflammatory benefits,** which helps to fight inflammation-related diseases such as asthma, irritable bowel syndrome and autoimmune disorders.

3. Intermittent fasting **relieves oxidative stress**, which is a key driver of ageing. Fasting increases a molecule that slows the ageing of arteries and skin.

4. Intermittent fasting can help with **insulin resistance and sensitivity**. It helps control blood sugar levels, which, in turn, helps with insulin complications that diabetic patients suffer from. Fasting may also lower the risk of developing diabetes.

5. Intermittent fasting **enhances fat burning,** especially around the waist. Belly fat can reduce by up to 7 per cent, or sometimes more, during fasting.

6. Intermittent fasting can **improve mental concentration** as well. During fasting, our brain produces a hormone that is good for mental functioning. This hormone is a protein called brain-derived neurotrophic factor (BDNF). An increase in BDNF helps improve focus and mental concentration.

7. Intermittent fasting **improves gut health** by decreasing blood sugar, reducing inflammation and encouraging fat burning. Along with the right foods, the microbes in the gut boost immune intolerance and tissue repair. Drinking lots of water during fasting enhances this benefit further. Hydration helps push away dysfunctional cells and clears the gut of bad bacteria.

8. Intermittent fasting **boosts the growth of good hormones**. The process of balanced hormone secretion contributes to numerous health benefits, such as cellular repair, fat burning and increased metabolism.

9. Intermittent fasting methods can lower blood pressure, triglycerides, cholesterol and LDL in the blood. This can **lower the risk of heart disease and improve heart health**.

However, intermittent fasting is not for everyone. It can also give you some side effects like:

1. **Irritability**: Irritability is very common during this period due to lack of food, especially if you are not used to it. Being hangry (anger borne out of hunger) is also a side effect some people experience during this period.

2. **Fatigue**: Lack of food can lead to low energy and fatigue.

3. **Slow reaction**: Low energy can lead to slow reactions to things and loss of interest.

4. **Dehydration**: Those who are not drinking enough liquids during this period can feel dehydrated.

If any of these side effects occur and persist for longer than three to four days, it is advisable to stop doing intermittent fasting.

Intermittent fasting can be uncomfortable for people with the following conditions:

1. Eating disorders

2. Amenorrhea

3. Pregnancy or breastfeeding

4. Low blood pressure

5. Being underweight

6. Diabetes

DR K'S PRO-TIP

My mantra for food is to eat what feels good tomorrow. Listen to your body's intuition. If you know that a burger will feel 'fun' now but tomorrow, you will feel heavy, don't eat it. Dessert every night might not be for you. You may experience increased sugar cravings, energy highs and lows, and dizziness and fainting if you don't eat sugar; these are not signs that your body loves or needs sugar but that there is an imbalance. Or maybe you are an emotional eater. When you are stressed, anxious, or bored and you turn to food, you are using food as a drug instead of as the nourishment it is. Be aware of your emotional trigger and recognize that food is not the solution.

Because of a lack of mindfulness and awareness, we move further and further away from what our body needs, and towards a never-ending cacophony of what people think and what the internet says. This confusion is only worsening this epidemic of poor eating. And it's time we end it and become mindful, 'lit' eaters!

7

SKINCARE AT HOME

Every patient post-lockdown has come to me with buckets of skincare issues and products bought after an errant Instagram advertisement binge. I see products from the US, UK, Europe, India, Korea, China – you name it, and it's there. The world has come to me in skincare products. And guess what, you all came to me despite that beauty stash, because it somehow didn't work.

Don't you wish you had saved that money instead? Yes, I wish you had too. And that you didn't dump hundreds of products on my desk that I have to now shame you into removing from your regime. Not fun. Instead, let me guide you on how to approach the whole process of buying skincare.

First, I will talk about how to intuitively care for your skin. Then I will break down the essentials and tell you what you should apply based on your age, and finally, I will go through the latest beauty trends and home devices. So, to invest in the right skincare, read on and learn what to keep and what to throw.

INTUITIVE SKINCARE

I am a believer in skinalism – skincare minimalism – and intuitive skincare. What is that? Intuitive skincare essentially means understanding your skin and choosing products according to what your skin wants. It is about intuitively understanding yourself.

If your skin feels oily, you'll use a more foaming face wash and maybe skip the moisturizer. If your skin feels dry, you might clean it with water or a micellar water or a cleansing oil, and use a heavy moisturizer. You'll change serums according to what you're looking for and even according to parts of your face. So, if your T-zone is oilier, maybe we'll use a serum that has salicylic acid, niacinamide, or green tea just for that area, to reduce oil. If maybe your cheeks are drier than usual, then you use a serum that has ceramides or omega-3 fatty acids for the drier parts of your face. The idea is to balance. You will use different things on different parts of your face, and change according to the time of day and the way your skin feels.

It is not about multi-product or multi-step routines. Intuitive skincare is the opposite of it. I do not like the ten-step Korean skincare routine. Indian skin was not designed to apply ten products on the face in the morning and at night. Essentially, it will clog your pores. Korean skin actually has fewer sebaceous glands and pores, so it can tolerate more products. Also, the weather is different from how it is here, with more pollution, population and dust. Not to mention the diversity of Indian skin types.

Intuitive skincare is a much better approach for Indian skin types as it is all about understanding yourself individually. Everybody's skin is different, everyone's lives are different, everyone's stress points are different. So, it is important that you choose your skincare according to you, not according to some mass-produced formula. Intuitive skincare will make your skin better because it's about you understanding what your skin needs and establishing a better relationship with it. And you can have a dermatologist or aesthetic specialist guide you, since you might not know the right answer to what your skin needs. That's what we're here for. But it's also a lot about you managing your skin at home as well. Nobody can understand your skin better than you can understand – if and when it feels oily, when it feels dry, and if your nose is the driest it's ever been.

It's different from a skin fast! Intuitive skincare is not the same thing as skin fasting because intuitive skincare may include serums, mists, toners, etc. It includes all of those products that you want for extra results, which, of course, might or might not be prescribed. However, a skin-fasting routine means simply doing nothing to your skin on a particular day. You will apply nothing on your face, or at most, a moisturizer and a sunblock. But you're taking a break from all actives. Technically, on a skin fast, you don't apply anything, but I do a modified skin fast where you still cleanse, moisturize and apply sunblock.

It is less wasteful! I think this approach should help us avoid beauty waste and hoarding more products (like the post-lockdown buckets you came to me with). Very often, we buy products because of sheer marketing. We're told that every product is some magical potion that's going to make us look like Zendaya, but that's not the case. That's why, if we have a better understanding of our skin, we'll end up wasting less money. We'll choose what we know or what we think will probably suit us.

It should ideally give you longer-lasting results, essentially because you're not throwing stuff on your face that isn't working for you: your skin will be more resilient, healthier and, overall, just better in the long term. If you're doing intuitive skincare, it's pretty much impossible to overdo it. Intuitive skincare also means stopping something when you feel you're overdoing it; it's about balance. Skinalism or intuitive skincare focuses on minimalism with results, thereby avoiding side effects. And nowadays, with cloth face masks, we have to cut down the layers to prevent maskne (mask-acne) too! The face masks increase pore obstruction and also irritation from actives due to occlusion of them, making them extra active, which can be harmful.

So how do you do intuitive skincare? Here are some easy rules to follow:

Don't double cleanse more than once a week if you have dry or sensitive skin. If you have oily skin, you can do this two to three times a week! Mists can be used always and at any time for anyone who has dehydrated skin, so it's an add-on that's safe for all. Avoid toners. If you must use one, get one in the form of an astringent or an AHA or BHA tonic, and use it no more than a few times a week. If you have sensitive skin, it's a no-no! Do not use an AHA and a retinoid/retinol on the same day unless prescribed by a doctor. Take a day off once a week from all actives for a skin fast. No more than one mask a week if you have actives such as AHAs, BHAs, retinols in your skincare regime. No home remedies if you are using the above actives in your skincare!

Remember, AHAs, BHAs, PHAs and retinols make your skin more sensitive because they remove the dead protective layer of keratin that sits on top of the skin. That's why the skin is brighter and less pigmented as it sheds the dead layer. Now with less protection, your skin is better but more sensitive.

So, you can't overdo it! Otherwise, you can end up with rashes because the barrier gets disrupted. Even rosacea can get triggered because of the excess barrier disruption.

Now you have the basics on how to add actives and create a skincare routine intuitively for your skin.

DR K'S PRO-TIPS

Let me introduce you to some new words in the skincare world (in case you haven't heard them yet! If you have: go pro!)

Multi-moisturizing

Choose different moisturizers for different parts of your face. Your dry cheeks need ceramides while your oily T-zone needs that niacinamide!

Multi-cleansing

Choose different cleansers for different areas of your face. For combination skin type, a foaming salicylic acid facewash for the T-zone and a cream- or milk-based one for the rest of the face that is normal to dry.

Skin fasting

A skin fast is basically an actives-free fast for a few days (up to forty days) to reset the acid mantle and epidermal barrier of the skin.

I like Sunday fasts for all active skincare and advise the same to my clients.

Sometimes, if I feel that products aren't working on my skin, I take a few weeks off. And if my skin still feels sensitive, I take a month off, and then restart my actives one by one.

CHOOSING YOUR BASICS

The foundation of your skincare regimen is cleanser, moisturizer and sunblock. Let me break it down on how to choose one for yourself. I promise you, it's not rocket science. Then, I will talk about skincare choices by age – what you should have and what you should throw out. First, let's talk about the ageless essentials.

Sunscreen

Ideally, a sunblock regimen should be introduced in childhood, but if you haven't started it young, start right now. It is the number one way to prevent pigmentation, tanning, wrinkles, ageing, pore enlargement, textural irregularities, freckles, and the list goes on. Wear it indoors and outdoors. Wear it when it's raining, when it's snowing, when you're crying, when you're talking on your cell phone (I am serious! Blue light blockers for your screen, guys! Your phone causes pigmentation and ageing, too, with all that blue light. It comes from your laptops and your screens. So, zinc oxide, a mineral sunblock ingredient, is a great agent to look for in your sunblock).

> **Quick tip**: Any mineral sunblock will help block the blue light from your sunscreens, so you don't need any special sunblock branding for blue light filtering.

Now, the most important question: How to choose the right sunblock?

Sometimes, you need to try ten or twenty different sunblock lotions or creams to find the one that makes your skin look normal, doesn't feel too greasy, and doesn't leave a grey cast or make you look too white. I prefer 100 per cent mineral sunblock as other chemical sunscreen agents can be absorbed into the bloodstream. The problem is that most people hate the white cast it leaves. However, I massage it in for ten minutes, and the white cast goes away. So that's my trick. All mineral sunscreens block blue light and visible light from overhead lighting too.

Titanium dioxide and zinc oxide are my favourite sunblock agents. They also block both UVA and UVB light. UVB light is that which tans you and can cause skin cancer. UVA light causes pigmentation, ageing, wrinkling, pore enlargement, and more. You want an SPF of 30 to 50 (more than that has only an incremental benefit while making the sunblock thicker and too greasy) for UVB protection, and UVA protection of PA++ at least (these measures are carried out by the skincare company through tests they have to complete on volunteers to show their level of efficacy).

What does SPF mean

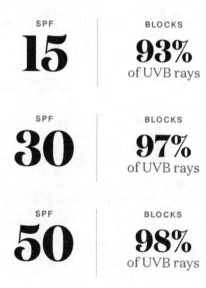

SPF	BLOCKS
15	**93%** of UVB rays
30	**97%** of UVB rays
50	**98%** of UVB rays

What's the benefit of each SPF?? See how there's only an improvement of 1 per cent in UVB protection by SPF 30 and SPF 50? You are only getting an extra 1 per cent of protection whilst requiring so much more sunscreen agents to increase the SPF. Yikes!

But SPF can't block 100 per cent of UVB rays and, in any case, how much UVB you get also depends on the quantity you use, how much you sweat and how much you reapply. SPF protects against tanning and skin cancer.

Another thing to look out for in your sunscreen is the PA rating, which is the protection grade against UVA rays and uses the Persistent Pigment Darkening scale at two to four hours of sun exposure.

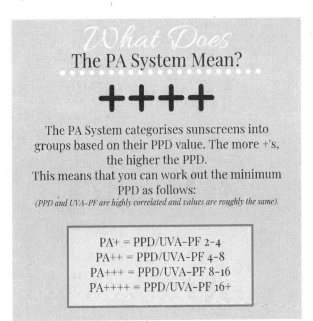

What Does The PA System Mean?

++++

The PA System categorises sunscreens into groups based on their PPD value. The more +'s, the higher the PPD.
This means that you can work out the minimum PPD as follows:
(PPD and UVA-PF are highly correlated and values are roughly the same).

PA+ = PPD/UVA-PF 2–4
PA++ = PPD/UVA-PF 4–8
PA+++ = PPD/UVA-PF 8–16
PA++++ = PPD/UVA-PF 16+

You typically want a PA ++ (moderate protection and above) for UVA protection and, even here, mineral sunblock agents are the best for protecting against UVAs.

Blue light

Nowadays, we don't need sunscreen just for the sun, but also for the light that our phones, laptops, tablet screens emit as we stare at them. This light is called blue light. Blue light is basically the emitted visible light between the wavelengths of 400 to 500 nm. The main source of blue light is sunlight, but digital screens, light-emitting diodes (LEDs), and fluorescent lighting serve as additional sources.

Just like sunlight, blue light in small controlled measures is helpful to the skin but with the kind of massive and continuous exposure we have all day, every day, it can be tremendously damaging.[55] Studies show that 'longer exposure to high-energy blue light can increase the amount of DNA damage, cell and tissue death, and injury, eye damage, skin barrier damage, and photoaging'. [56]

Now for those that wear sunblock religiously and still see freckles, sun spots, pigmentation and early ageing, it is likely due to HEV or high energy visible light, which is high emission like the blue light from your phones and screens. This light penetrates 50 per cent more than UVA rays and creates more free radicals that cause cellular damage. So, your screens are actually killing your skin. Again, mineral sunblock to the rescue!

Use two full fingers worth for the face and neck. Don't forget your chest, arms, back, and legs: these get cumulative sun exposure and show unnecessary skin effects later on. Reapply every four hours whether you are indoors or outdoors.

And I will say it again: wear sunblock! Every day, all day.

Face cleanser and moisturizer

Face cleansers (or washes) and moisturizers are the very basics of your skincare at home. At the very least, you need to have clean and hydrated skin every day. Using intuitive skincare here as well, here are some pointers on how to select face cleansers and moisturizers as per your skin's needs.

How to choose your face wash or cleanser:

- pH balanced (pH should be around 5.5). If pH is too high, like with any soap, it'll cause dryness, irritation, allergy, and more, so no soap.

- Evaluate on your skin. If your skin feels dry after using a certain cleanser, use a gentler cream/oil-based cleanser or a micellar water. If skin feels oily, then one with more foam is okay.

- Choose different cleansers for morning and night. Your skin may feel oilier at night and drier in the morning.

- If you're looking for glow, use an AHA- or PHA-based cleanser with a pH of 3.5-4.5. This will boost skin renewal and help impart a glow. Ideally, use only at night because it makes you more likely to tan otherwise.

How to choose your moisturizer:

- If your skin feels oily, you don't need to use a moisturizer at all. But if you feel like you still want one, use a gel-based one.

- For acne-prone skin, moisturizers designed for acne-prone skin that are light and oil-free are key.

- For dry skin look for heavier creams with ceramides, waxes and stronger barrier agents.

- Change your moisturizer based on the time of day. If in the day you feel too greasy because of sunblock, use a lighter lotion or gel. And at night, use a heavier one.

- Multi-moisturizing, use different moisturizers for different parts of your face, especially if you have combination skin.

- My favourite trick: SLUGGING. Apply Vaseline petroleum jelly to your full face or neck or any area that feels dry after you apply your moisturizer that has a strong humectant in it such as glycerine, hyaluronic acid (HA), sodium lactate or polyglutamic acid or urea. Leave it on overnight. Watch how moisturized your skin is the next day! (No, it does not usually cause acne; just don't do it more than once a week.)

TREND ALERT: MOISTURE SANDWICH FOR EXTRA HYDRATION

If your skin is having an especially dry day, try a moisture sandwich:

- Cleanse your face or spritz with a mist so that your skin is damp.

- Then apply a hydrating serum (on damp skin) that has humectants, which bind water and bring it into the skin.

- Then, immediately apply something occlusive (Vaseline jelly), a butter (shea butter), or beeswax to hold in all that moisture you bound from the damp water from your skin and the humectant.

HOW TO READ A SKINCARE LABEL

It is hard to read a skincare label and not feel lost. Let me break down how to know what you are getting, so that you don't feel lost at a beauty counter.

Step 1: Identify your skincare active

Ideally, you already know which active you want, and now you are looking at the percentage at which it is present in your skincare. Hopefully, the company already makes it clear to you on the marketing information, but in case they don't, look at how high up it is in the ingredient list. If it's one of the first few, it's in a decent percentage. If it's all the way at the end, it's barely there.

Step 2: Will the product work?

See if any studies were done on the product involving real people. If they were, amazing! You are in the clear. Typically this information would be on the brand's website or on the box of the product itself. The brand will make that information readily available to you, don't worry. If not, were any studies done on the actives? And if that's also not there, you will have to do some serious sleuthing online to find out from reviews how well that ingredient works.

Step 3: Check the pH

Some products will inform you that they are pH balanced to the skin. For cleansers, washes or soaps without AHAs, PHAs, or BHAs, that is awesome, but otherwise, it's not really necessary to know this information. Only soaps or washes will have out-of-range pH that can irritate the skin. The other products, such as home peels, or AHA/BHA/PHA-related ingredients or even vitamin C, need a lower pH than the skin to be more effective. Here, the pH won't be mentioned.

Step 4: Does it have artificial fragrance in it?

I tend to avoid products with artificial fragrances in them because the company is not obliged to label all the individual ingredients that are in a perfume or fragrance due to intellectual property. But I find these very fragrances can possibly be allergenic or irritating in skincare. So, if it says 'Fragrance' or 'Parfum', chances are it's chock-full of artificial fragrance.

Step 5: Understand the PAO

The PAO is the period after opening, so if it only has six months after opening, that's something you should know and keep in mind. I often label the product with the date I opened it or the date I think it expires to keep myself from the risk of using an expired product.

8

SKINCARE BY THE DECADE

Now that we have covered the eternal basics, let's see what our skin needs and wants at different ages of our lives. Our skin's needs change as we grow, and we need to ensure we keep up with that change. Don't worry, I have you covered! With all that is essential and non-essential in every decade. So, just follow my lead.

> ### DR K'S PRO-TIP
>
> We spend most of our time focusing on our faces, but our necks, chests (decollete), and hands get ignored and they tend to reveal the signs of ageing first. Apply the same skincare to those areas if you can, and don't forget your sunblock either.

TWENTIES

The twenties are a time for adulting. And serious adulting requires serious skincare. First of all, by the age of twenty-five, your body will start degrading more collagen than it makes and will lose approximately 1 per cent collagen every year. This is also the time where pigmentation, freckles and some pore enlargement will start to show.

For some reason, every twenty-something has products from *The Ordinary*. Okay, that's great, I'm glad it's cheap and quick, but we really need to distil down what ingredients you actually need, as opposed to buying into every skincare active trend.

Essential ingredients:

- Vitamin C (ideally with ferulic acid as the combo is much more effective)
- Bakuchiol: If you have acne, or tend to get acne, and also want an anti-ageing boost, bakuchiol is a great new active out there that can help boost collagen, while reducing acne. However, you should note that there is not enough data on it at the moment to consider it equal to or more effective than retinol, but it has been shown to boost collagen, and it's not irritating, so yay!

How to choose the right vitamin C product

This is what you need to look for on the label:

- Look for at least 8 per cent vitamin C (ascorbic acid); greater than 20 per cent is not required. More than 20 per cent can cause irritation, so be careful! More does not mean good.

- To get effective results from your vitamin C cream/serum, and good penetration of L-ascorbic acid, the pH must be below 4.2. That's why adding ferulic acid is great because it brings the pH down to about 3.5.

- Some other vitamin C options include ascorbyl 6-palmitate, tetra-iso palmitoyl ascorbate, magnesium ascorbyl phosphate, sodium ascorbyl phosphate, ascorbyl 2-glucoside, ascorbyl 2-phosphate-6-palmitate, and 3-O-ethyl ascorbate. Yes, those are difficult names but can be useful to know. Ascorbyl 6-palmitate, ascorbyl-2-glucoside, and tetra-iso palmitoyl ascorbate demonstrate, to a greater or lesser extent, superior stability and greater ease of formulation. Ascorbyl 2-glucoside is one of the most important L-ascorbic acid derivatives, because of its resistance to reduction and oxidation. It is also easily degraded by a-glucosidase to release L-ascorbic acid and glucose.

- If you are acne-prone, do not use serums. Keep it to fluids, as propylene glycol is well known to trigger zits, as can other agents that help solubilize vitamin C into serums. Use a fluid instead. If you are dry skinned, vitamin C Oil is also amazing.

Non-essentials, or optional ingredients:

- Retinol: I know it's a buzzword for anti-ageing, but let's keep that to your thirties or at least your late twenties. It can dry you out and make your skin more sensitive. For your twenties, your lifestyle is rough enough.

- Niacinamide: While it can reduce oil secretion, and is mildly anti-ageing, it is non-essential. Yes, I know it is also a buzzword ingredient, but it's not the main event of your skincare regime. Your vitamin C and your sunblock are. Remember that!

THIRTIES

Your thirties are your time to thrive and arrive! And your skincare needs to take care of you and the changes you will go through in this important decade of your life.

As you traverse your thirties, you see enlarged pores, fine lines, and textural irregularity coming around to play, and even early traces of sagging can be seen. Those laugh lines aren't as laughable now! Freckles and pigmentation start appearing, or worsening, and this is typically the age when most people say they notice a lot more pigmentation around their chin and forehead.

This is also when I tend to see a lot of neck lines popping up, along with some neck sagging. If you have more than one centimetre of pinchable skin in this area, it's time to get cracking!

> ### DR K'S PRO-TIP
>
> Neck lines and neck sagging are showing up earlier than before, and I believe it's due to TECH NECK – the sagging that happens because we are constantly looking down at our phones. Keep your head up when using your smartphone, and your skin will thank you.

Essential Ingredients:

- Vitamin C, ferulic acid (strong antioxidant)
- Moisturizer
- Sunblock
- Retinol (boosts collagen, as net collagen in the body decreases from the age of approximately twenty-five)

HOW TO USE A RETINOL

- Apply at night. Start alternate nights or a couple of times a week and do the retinol sandwich: moisturize – retinol – moisturize.

- Use a pea-sized amount for the entire face, not more than that. Also, apply on dry skin to prevent stinging. Or you can mix retinol with your moisturizer and apply. You can even apply it for one or two hours, and then wash it off.

- Build up from a couple of times a week to nearly every day. But make sure to take a skin fast at least once a week. Retinol boosts collagen, but it can make your skin more sensitive and reduce the keratin layer that protects the epidermis. So, if you overdo it, you can give yourself a rash. To get results while keeping the skin safe, take a break once a week.

- AHA/PHA: At this age, our skin renewal slows down too, so it's a good time to add in alpha-hydroxy acids or polyhydroxy acids to your skincare for extra skin renewal and glow. But start alternate nights with the retinol – don't use both together as then, the keratin layer becomes too thin and the epidermal barrier too weak.

WHAT ARE AHA/ PHAS? AND WHAT IS THE DIFFERENCE BETWEEN THEM?

AHAs are small to large acids that stimulate the exfoliation of skin cells. Derived from sugar, glycolic acid is the most common of these and can even help with pigmentation. It is commonly used in chemical peels. However, since it is small, it can be irritating as it gets absorbed easily into the skin. Lactic acid is a gentler AHA found in buttermilk, and it is also hydrating. Now, polyhydroxy acids are gentler versions of AHAs: they are essentially chemical exfoliants that are designed to be gentle and non-irritating. They exfoliate dead skin, make skin more even toned, and also impart brightness. Nearly everyone can use it, except for those who spend a lot of time in the sun, because it makes you sensitive to the sun. But, it won't be as effective as glycolic acid. That is because PHAs are a much larger molecule, so they can't penetrate as deeply as glycolic acid can. So, they won't work as much on pigmentation either. However, you can use them regularly, with minimal risks. They are ideal for dry, sensitive skin.

Consider using PHAs as a cleanser for extra brightening or in your face cream with a good SPF.

Non-essential ingredients:

- Hyaluronic acid: Needed more when your skin gets drier as you approach pre-menopause.

- Polyglutamic acid: Similar to HA, only needed for extremely dry skin.

WHAT IS POLYGLUTAMIC ACID?

Polyglutamic acid is derived from fermented soybeans: it is a water-soluble peptide that is non-toxic, biodegradable and safe for the skin. It binds water like hyaluronic acid does and can, in fact, retain almost five times as much moisture as HA. So, if your skin is dehydrated, and you want it to be more supple and your wrinkles to look less prominent, a highly moisture-binding ingredient is a must. It also prohibits the destruction of HA, by inhibiting the action of hyaluronidase, so it is anti-ageing too! As we all know, HA is always present in the skin and helps bind water so that the skin remains supple, hydrated and young. Regarding polyglutamic acid, so far, no real side effects have been reported, although there is always a risk of idiopathic irritation or allergy. If you are allergic to soybeans, you cannot use it. Regarding PGA, we can't say it is better than HA yet, but in the lab, it does bind more water. However, there are way more studies on HA, so wait for more data!

I make sure I use a heavy moisturizer as the top-most layer to bind the water that is attracted to the PGA and HA in the skin, so it doesn't leak out. Apply a barrier-enhancing moisturizer on top of that super strong humectant. And if you can't afford PGA, then just get simple glycerine. It is a powerful humectant too.

FORTIES

Forties are an important decade as most women enter the premenopausal stages at this time. It can affect your skin in several ways, so your skincare is of utmost important in this decade.

In your forties, you will see lines, sagging and enlarged pores becoming much more prominent, and even some jowls, neck loosening and a mild double chin can start showing. You can expect those freckles and pigmentation to only get worse from here. Also, as you hit premenopause, the skin will start to change with your changing hormones. Your skin may become drier or you may begin to get zits around your periods.

Essential ingredients:

- Vitamin C
- Ferulic acid
- Barrier-based moisturizers: sunblock, retinol
- Peptides
- Hyaluronic acid

WHAT IS HYALURONIC ACID?

Hyaluronic acid is a humectant that binds water and also boosts collagen. But you have to be careful with it as some low-molecular-weight HAs can trigger irritation or worsen sensitivity and rosacea. So, you need to look for those that are suitable for rosacea-prone skin. All HAs are not made equal. Usually, they are a combo of LMW (low molecular weight) and HMW (high molecular weight), and the more expensive ones are usually better. LMW hyaluronic acid absorbs into the skin and will bind water and increase the moisturization within it as any good humectant does. Because rosacea is so easy to trigger, some LMW hyaluronic acids will trigger rosacea. But HMW hyaluronic acid will sit on top of the skin, form a barrier and protect it, thus, proving anti-inflammatory.

WHAT ARE PEPTIDES?

Peptides are anti-ageing ingredients, typically messenger molecules that stimulate fibroblasts to increase collagen. Basically, for your cells to make collagen, they need a signal to turn on. The peptides are those signals. Unlike retinol, they are not irritating, not drying, and they don't make your skin sensitive to the sun, so you can combine them with anything.

Non-essential ingredients:

- Vitamin B5: This is simply a moisturizing agent called panthenol. Do not get sucked in. It's already present in nearly every product.

- Vitamin E: It's an antioxidant, but your skincare is already enough with vitamin C and ferulic acid. Besides, vitamin E can sometimes cause allergy or acne.

FIFTIES AND BEYOND

This is when menopause hits you and ageing starts to accelerate. Oestrogen is an anti-ageing hormone and, once you hit menopause, the active form of oestrogen takes a dive. Sagging, lines and dry skin become prominent.

Essential ingredients:

- Vitamin C

- Ferulic acid

- Hyaluronic acid/polyglutamic acid

- Ceramides: At this age, your skin barrier becomes weaker and the glue that keeps skin together comprises ceramides and humectants such as natural moisturizing factors. Add those ceramides back into your skin to combat the dryness.

- Emollients (Less testosterone and less active oestrogen will cause more dryness for women, and less testosterone for men will also make skin drier). Emollients help keep the skin moist with ingredients such as light liquid paraffin and shea butter.

- Sunblock

- Retinol

- Peptides

Non-essential ingredients:

I love facial oils for this age group, but they aren't essential:

- Rosehip oil

- Grapeseed oil

- Coconut oil, if not too acne-prone

- Hemp seed oil: It has omega-3, omega-6, and omega-9 fatty acids, which are great for moisturization.

MYTHBUSTER

All hemp has CBD, which is calming for the skin.
Truth:

Hemp seed oil is made from the seed of the hemp plant, while hemp oil is made from the leaves, the stalk, etc.

Hemp seed oil does not contain CBD (cannabidiol), but it can have up to 0.3 per cent THC legally (THC is what makes you high from marijuana), which is so low it's almost negligible. But hemp oil can have both CBD and THC in it.

CBD oil helps improve mood, anxiety and pain, and when applied topically, it can help in inflammation-related skin issues too. But sometimes, it can worsen rosacea. Studies are still on to gauge the effectiveness of CBD on specific skin conditions.

GENERAL AREAS OF CONCERN

Under-eye skincare

Under-eye is an area of constant concern, most of the time regardless of age. There are amazing therapies that can help you minimize dark circles (depending on their nature), and I will talk about them in the next chapter. But there is a lot you can do in your home skincare routines as well to improve their appearance.

Let's understand what causes **dark circles** and how to treat them by targeting the root problem. The causes can be separated into four main categories.

1   **Genes**. If someone in your family has had dark circles and you've had them for a long time, it's likely that your genes are the problem. While it's easy to blame your genes for your under-eye woes, it's vital to know what exactly it is that is genetically transmitted. Many people, anatomically,

have deep-set eyes, which means that the eye socket is recessed or set back in the skull. Instead of a smooth line between the eye bone and the cheekbone, the eye bone is deeper back, resulting in a hollow that causes a shadow to appear, making the under-eye area look darker. This particular cause is actually easy to treat – simply fill the hollow! While no cream can do this, simple treatments such as natural platelet-rich plasma or HA fillers can be injected into the area to fill the space, thereby eradicating the shadow and the under-eye circles. Learn more about the benefits and side effects of these treatments in the next chapter!

2. **Pigmentation**. If a person has a tendency for this area to get discoloured, it makes them look tired perpetually, even though they may be well rested. It's simply that the skin has a tendency to create more melanin in that area, resulting in dark discolouration. Sometimes, friction from rubbing your eyes and sun exposure can worsen this. Luckily, it is treatable. First things first, start wearing sunblock whether you are indoors or outdoors. This will prevent further darkening from UV rays. Next, apply anti-pigmentation creams containing actives such as kojic acid, alpha-arbutin or liquorice extract. These gentle ingredients will help remove pigment from this extra-sensitive area. Finally, for when the pigment just won't go, consider lasers such as Clearlift, or simple metabolic peels.

3. **Poor blood circulation and lymphatic flow**. These are the type of dark circles that appear when you don't sleep

enough and wake up all puffy. This is pretty easy to treat and can be done simply at home. Importantly, you must make sure you get enough rest. Also, do not consume salt after 8 p.m. so that excess salt is removed from your system. Some home remedies are also very convenient and can be done in a few minutes, especially before a big day. The most handy and effective among all the remedies is using cold tea bags that we mentioned in chapter 4 on DIY skincare. Regarding skincare, consider including ingredients such as hesperidin and vitamin K. Hesperidin is an active that helps improve blood flow and reduce inflammation.

4. **Ageing.** Now last but not the least, let's not forget the most common cause of under-eye circles, i.e., ageing. As the human body ages, collagen production becomes less, making our tissues weaker and saggier. This creates a hollow while also allowing fluid to accumulate in the area and lines to form. Luckily, this is manageable. In skincare, we want retinol and peptides to be added to our routine. But to be honest, it's mostly preventative and won't solve the issue. While plastic surgery is an option, for those who don't want to go under the knife, treatments such as Ulthera and Under Eye Rescue or under-eye radiofrequency are designed to increase collagen synthesis.

DR K'S PRO-TIP

DO NOT RUB YOUR EYES! It will make them dry, irritated and pigmented. I am serious: I once treated a patient's under-eye circles with the help of anti-inflammatory creams to fix the rash she got from rubbing her eyes too much. Needless to say, she had to stop rubbing her eyes too. Nine hundred rupees and a few months of good habits, and voila!

Best ingredients for under-eye skincare

Do not use the same products on your face and under the eyes. The under-eye skin is thinner than your normal skin, so you can't use the same actives or in the same way as the rest of your face.

- Vitamin C brightens and prevents oxidative damage, and also helps with pigmentation.
- Retinol boosts collagen.
- Peptides also boost collagen.

These are my favourites for any brightening or anti-ageing benefits. You can use light moisturizers in addition to these. Some other actives helpful for pigmentation in the under-eye area are alpha-arbutin, kojic acid or liquorice extract.

Only under-eye creams will not always be able to solve your problems. They can help a little, but if you have the Grand Canyon under your beautiful eyes, no cream will do the job. That's where treatments come in.

Lips

I get many patients who complain of dark or dry lips, and they are actually pretty common.

Why do lips get dark?

Sun exposure, eczema, repetitive rubbing, licking or smacking of lips, smoking, artificial colours in our makeup and just plain old genes can cause lip darkening. Unfortunately, there are no products or ingredients that particularly work in reducing lip pigmentation, although ingredients such as alpha-arbutin and kojic acid can be used. But the most important thing to do is to wear sunblock and use a good lip balm while avoiding irritants. I would also choose a completely natural lipstick that uses natural pigments instead of traditional lipstick brands. Refer to p. 163, where I discuss how to read product labels.

Why do lips get dry?

Besides internal dehydration (drink more water, obviously!), lip dehydration is common, and licking your lips will make them even drier! I know that sounds crazy but every time you lick your lips, that liquid evaporates along with water within the lips, making you feel dry so you lick your lips again, and it becomes a terrible vicious cycle. Stop licking your lips! It's not sexy! It makes your lips chapped and rough and terribly unkissable.

Instead, every time you want to touch, rub, or lick your lips, pull out a trusty lip balm with SPF in it, and apply. And don't pull off the skin. Never!

Favourite Skincare Cocktails

This is a great part of home skincare. Let me show you how to mix your actives in a beauty cocktail that improves results and saves time! Best for those on the go. These babies are the martinis, mimosas and margaritas of your skincare: delicious and effective for your skin!

- **Vitamin C + Hyaluronic Acid**: Vitamin C protects the skin from antioxidant damage, while hyaluronic acid improves the moisture levels of the skin. High MW hyaluronic acid creates a stronger skin barrier.

- **Vitamin C + Arbutin**: Vitamin C brightens the skin, while arbutin helps to reduce pigmentation while also brightening the skin.

- **Vitamin C + Sunscreen**: I like this combo because vitamin C helps with UV protection, and sunblock is the ultimate for UV protection. But you still need a separate vitamin C with a higher percentage, because with sunblock you need to use two tablespoons every four hours.

- **Retinol + Hyaluronic Acid**: Retinol boosts collagen synthesis and increases cellular turnover and is anti-ageing. Hyaluronic acid improves moisture retention, so it helps prevent retinol-induced dryness, while also being anti-ageing and creating a healthier skin barrier.

- **Retinol + Peptides**: Both retinol and peptides are anti-ageing actives, and boost collagen synthesis synergistically.

- **AHAs + Kojic Acid**: AHAs induce cellular renewal, improve glow and help with pigmentation. Kojic acid works to increase glow and improve pigmentation.

Using masks at home

It is good to use masks at home once in a while but be careful. Figure out what you need and don't overdo it.

Masking essentials:

- You should use masks no more than one to two times a week.

- Do not combine any mask containing actives for brightening or anti-ageing with an AHA, PHA, BHA or retinol the same day. You can irritate your skin by doing so.

- Don't do it before you bleach, or you will give yourself a rash.

- I HATE SHEET MASKS! Please don't use them. The results last for like one hour. And they are bad for the environment. And they don't work. Even the rubber masks are not much better.

I prefer peel-off and wash-off masks or leave-on masks. When you are looking for masks, think about what result you want or what skin issue you want to temporarily address, and then choose accordingly.

When looking for:
- Brightening masks – Look for ones with AHAs, PHAs.
- Anti-acne – Look for ones with BHAs, sulphur, AHAs, clays.
- Hydrating – Look for ones with humectants: urea, glycerine, HA, barrier agents such as petrolatum, paraffin, waxes, butters.

CAUTION

SKINCARE BUFFS – Those of you who want every active ever created on your face on a daily basis, you will end up at my door six months later with rosacea, meaning your skin will be super sensitive, irritated, and it will feel like nothing will work. Please start with one active at a time. Be intuitive, notice if your skin feels sensitive or there's too much sensation, or you are tanning too quickly. And DO YOUR SKIN FASTS without fail!

ESSENTIAL HOME DEVICES

Another helpful element in your intuitive home skincare is home devices. There is a range of devices that you can use at home for when you need that much-needed boost but cannot make it out (or there is a lockdown – not an uncommon possibility these days). I am here to guide you through how you can buy the best and use them in an effective way.

Home LED masks

Home LED masks are great for treating acne, boosting collagen, and improving wound healing. They operate on the concept of low-level biostimulation, so they emit a low-level light to stimulate the skin. You must get one that is US FDA-approved, because if the power of light is too much, you aren't getting the benefit. It has to be a perfectly titrated power of light. Don't risk your skin to save a few bucks. You don't want burns, you want a glow.

LED hair helmets

The LED light results in biostimulation, which is also proven to increase hair growth. There are many brands available but ensure you buy US FDA approved. You really want to do this regularly for at least three to six months. It's super convenient because you can watch Netflix or play with your kids while the helmet is on your head, and you will literally be preventing hair fall and boosting hair growth at the same time! It's a safe and beneficial use of time. Whenever I have hair fall, I start popping iron and putting my LED hair helmet on. In one month, my scalp responds.

Gua Sha massage

It's great for improved lymphatic drainage and can help your face look a bit firmer. Go for a Gua Sha that feels right for you (different crystals have different properties or energies but I am not an expert on crystals, so I leave that to your research and discretion). I recommend doing this a few times a week, but if you have rosacea, drop it to once a week.

Microcurrent devices

Using electric stimulation, these devices force the muscles to contract, resulting in improved facial appearance. They can help tighten your facial muscles to make your face look more toned. Buy a good one, and do it as per the instructions. I would recommend using it at least once a week if you can, because your face can really respond well to this facial muscle toning, and it's great to do at home.

NON-ESSENTIAL DEVICES TO THROW AWAY

Much like skincare products, there has been a proliferation of skincare devices as well. While we talked about the ones we need, here are some popular ones that I don't consider very useful and, certainly, not essential, even though they do work on occasion and are good to use once in a while. But some of these I want you to do a burning ceremony for.

Face rollers: These increase the efficacy of your skincare but by very little. There is no real benefit and a higher risk of irritation for your skin.

Ice globes/ice rollers: If you want a quick glow or want your face to look a little less red or inflamed, or your pores to be tighter for an hour, it's fine. Long-term benefit is negligible.

Home exfoliating devices: This is not required and can cause excessive irritation if overdone. A normal scrub is enough!

Face massager: Don't waste your time. It does nothing more than what a regular massage can do.

THROW THESE OUT FOR SURE

Home derma-rollers or microneedling devices: Please don't do this. You will give yourself scars that cannot be reversed. These should be done properly by medical professionals.

Home laser hair-removal devices: They don't work. They don't work. They don't work. And there is a risk of burns, and of even increasing the hair growth in the area instead of reducing it. Please don't do this. I beg you! That money could be spent way better on a wonderful anti-ageing cream.

After reading all these tips, you must be thinking, 'Okay, now I will do my skincare and use my home devices, but will that solve all my skin problems?' You know what, it will solve a lot of them. It will make your skin significantly healthier, brighter, stronger and way more resilient (it will also do the same for your bank balance). Over time, you will also be able to prevent a lot of issues you otherwise may have faced earlier on, or issues that could have become terribly severe. If you want to test this, try treating one arm and leave the other arm untreated. Or do half and half of your neck (this might look weird, so you may want to stick to the arms). Watch the difference between the two areas over the next six months. That's really all the proof you need!

Now what to do for the rest of your problems? And what about all those awesome treatments for which you keep seeing 'before and afters' on Instagram? Don't worry, I am going to guide you there too. Read on to learn about the best treatments for your concerns.

9

FINISHING TOUCH

You are gorgeous just as you are, and I always believe that. I map out all my treatments keeping that belief in mind: my job is to make the best in you shine and glow! If your skin feels good, and your skincare is on point, sure, treatments may not be required. But let me tell you, no cream or scrub will erase blackheads, and nothing can prevent all the sun and pollution damage all of us are accruing every day. That damage is worsening the ageing process, increasing pigmentation and pores, and reducing the vitality of your skin. So, good skin upkeep is essential with the current environmental degradation.

I know it is hard to navigate what treatments to go for when there is a deluge of information and no clarity. I'm going to break it down for you into three categories: **prevention, correction, maintenance**. Wherever you are, whichever clinic you are in, you want to know what category the treatment is in, and how effective it will be for your specific concerns. First, let's discuss what I mean by prevention, correction, and maintenance and why they are important.

Prevention and 'Youngering': As the famous saying goes, prevention is better than cure! We all know we are going to age, so why not try to prevent its damaging effects by doing what I love to call 'youngering'?

Correction: Maybe there is a part of your skin or face that doesn't make you feel beautiful. You don't feel like you are in your own skin. Scars, acne, wrinkles – I can understand. If this is you, what you need are some correction treatments.

Maintenance: Once you feel like you have the skin you want and life is good, remember – all good things need to be maintained.

DR K'S PRO-TIP

There are three layers of your skin:

Top layer: Has issues of dullness, tanning, some freckles, some pigmentation.

Second layer: Can have issues of wrinkles, pigmentation, freckles, pores, scars.

Third layer: Can have issues of sagging, deep lines, some scars.

Therapies that cover all three layers or combos of therapies for all three layers are the most rejuvenating because all your skin concerns are covered. So keep that in mind!

Now, let's talk about these in detail and you can pick the ones you most identify with. Also, do note that I list here treatments that I offer, but some form of these should be available at the clinic you are consulting. It may have a different name, so check the procedures, companies and ingredients, and you should be on your way! To help you with this, after every few treatments, I have added notes on 'what to look for in your city' when trying to find these. Let's start with 'youngering' or preventing as much skin damage as possible.

PREVENTION

I am a big believer in youngering. What is youngering? It's a process that makes your skin actually younger, not just look younger. We want that same baby collagen, suppleness, glow and skin strength or, at least, keep it as youthful as possible, right? We also want our skin cells to behave like they did when we were younger! Remember as teenagers, if we got a cut, the mark would just disappear? That stops happening in our twenties, and then marks and long-lasting marks become a part of life. So we also want our skin to improve its behaviour overall. There are several therapies that can work for 'youngering' you. Let's talk about them.

Microneedling

Consider microneedling, which basically means boosting the same collagen you had as a baby; it's essentially reversing time. Small micro-needles are used to create micro-channels in the skin, and serums are simultaneously injected into the skin tissues through these channels (don't worry, it's not too many needles, you don't even feel it). This encourages the skin to produce baby collagen – the collagen we produce in our early childhood days, which is super effective for healing. This baby collagen is better than the wound collagen that is produced after an injury and is more resilient, supple and elastic. Microneedling will further improve the behaviour of keratinocytes and melanocytes when trauma such as scratches, burns or rashes or zits happen, and also reduce marks and pigmentation gradually! We do it at the right depth of 0.5 mm, which is at the junction of the dermis and epidermis, with the right endpoint and the right ingredients (you can't use home skincare for microneedling, as you need special products. They have to be without fragrance, colour, certain preservatives, certain solubilizers and more – otherwise, they can cause irritation and acne).

Two microneedling treatments that I love and offer are Good Genes Therapy and the Infuse Me facial.

Good Gene Therapy uses a vacuum-based rolling device that first requires exfoliation, for an even skin surface. Then, the machine ensures even deposition of the product beneath the skin through the vacuum, and it is followed up with collagen-boosting LED. It's a more titrated and scientific way of performing microneedling. It is best suited for you if you want glowing, healthy skin and laser-like results, but may have a lot of sun exposure in your life or you don't feel comfortable with lasers. It is also a great base therapy for any good preventative regime. It is Youngering 101! It works best for rejuvenation, hydration, glow, pores, lines and more. Good Gene Facial is the most effective, pain-free delivery of essential nutrients to the skin. It's effective for all skin conditions such as rosacea, pigmentation, pores, even acne. I would not do it on actively rashy or irritated skin, or with any ingredient you are allergic to.

The Infuse Me facial is simply basic microneedling, and is probably available at most centres around India. So, if you just want to get started and don't need as much nourishment or drastic results, or it is your first baby step into skincare, then basic microneedling is for you. It is best suited for you if you have dryness, pigmentation, textural issues or large pores and want clear baby-soft skin. We use a microneedling skin pen to create small channels in the skin that help us infuse serums and actives as per your skin concern (glow, pigmentation, anti-ageing, hydration). Because the microneedling pen also creates small, invisible injuries on the skin surface, it triggers the production of collagen to heal from the trauma. The result is glowing, supple and younger-looking skin that everyone will want to touch!

PRP

You should consider PRP for *youngering* your skin. PRP is Platelet Rich Plasma, which involves drawing your blood, treating it and injecting it back into your skin after activating your natural collagen boosters in it. Let me tell you about PRP or the 'Vampire facelift'.

PRP, or the Vampire Facelift, is for you if you want a completely natural way to tackle those ageing signs. PRP involves drawing your blood, treating it in the clinic, and injecting the growth factors of blood plasma back into your skin to boost collagen production by activating stem cells.

This is super effective in healing under-eye circles, fine lines and lack of elasticity and glow almost immediately, with long-lasting results. It's FDA-approved and a very safe way of solving almost every age-related skin issue, including dry and rough skin.

Skin Boosters

This is the ultimate *youngering* treatment! Skin boosters are the newest innovation in injectable treatments to enter the Indian market. Profhilo and other skin boosters, such as Juvederm Volite and Restylane Vitale, are designed to hydrate your skin from the deeper layers and stimulate collagen production naturally. They are bio-remodelers, which make use of stabilized hyaluronic acid to actually remodel multiple layers of your skin. Juvederm Volite and Restylane Vitale work on a more superficial layer to achieve more dewy skin, while Profilho works on deeper layers to also add elasticity and suppleness, and a little natural lift through deep hydration. Skin boosters are a way to make your skin youthful, truly lit and plump from within. Here's everything you need to know about them.

How do skin boosters work?

Skin boosters are unlike other injectable treatments, differing from dermal fillers. Hyaluronic acid can be used in serums, in fillers, in supplements and now, also in biostimulators when used in the right proportion.

This works directly on the source of the skin (deeper layers) that's causing ageing, as opposed to superficially attempting to reverse signs of ageing.

One type of skin booster, Profilho,[57] claims that it stimulates the fibroblast cells, thereby increasing collagen and elastin production; activates the keratinocytes to increase the synthesis of collagen and elastin; and preserves and encourages the viability of adipocytes that affect the quality of adipose tissue.

While a filler is designed to fill your skin as the name suggests, Profhilo is designed to stimulate and hydrate your skin from within the deeper layers.

Benefits of skin boosters

The reason I choose skin boosters is that it makes 'reversing time' with your skin possible, and I love that! For youngering your skin, you want lots of collagen and elastin. You want the adipocytes to behave like younger skin, not depleted like in older skin. You want deep hydration and suppleness. Skin boosters enable your skin to work harder and faster, as it did when it was younger, instead of making a superficial difference. It's truly a hardworking injectable that works on the principle of youngering your skin with every session, giving it the capability to reverse signs of ageing and make you appear younger.

Do you need it? If your skin is lacking lustre, hydration, tautness or just feeling limp, and is aged and lifeless on the whole, skin boosters are the perfect treatment for you. While we often see an immediate lift (with deeper boosters, not the more superficial ones) and glow, over the next few weeks after your procedure, there is a boost in skin dewiness, suppleness and elasticity as well.

Younger clients end up with a sort of indescribable feeling about looking better and just can't put a finger on why they are looking perkier. For older clients (above thirty-five), I tend to use Profilho, as they often see more of a visible lift, although some have deeper dehydration and collagen loss and may need more sessions to treat those concerns.

For younger clients, I prefer Juvederm Volite or Restylane Skin Boosters – because they don't lack elasticity but often just need superficial hydration that no cream can manage to give due to the lifestyles we all lead. So for that dewy effect, the more superficial skin boosters are helpful. Sometimes, I combine both together for extra deep and superficial boosting; and I add PRP sometimes, too!

SKIN BOOSTERS VS DERMAL FILLERS

Are you deciding between skin boosters and dermal fillers? Here's what you need to know:

- While dermal fillers structure the face, plump up lips, lift the skin and visibly improve the appearance of signs of ageing, skin boosters works on healing and remodelling the skin from within, genuinely making it younger and healthier as opposed to superficially filling it in.

- Skin boosters make your skin healthier and assist it in regenerating better, the way it did in your youth. It will result in reduced need for fillers in the future through its preventative effect.

- Both types of injectables are made with 100 per cent hyaluronic acid, which is bio-compatible, bringing the risk factor associated with it down to almost nil.

- Fillers can be used for younger and older clients to solve a problem or for facial reshaping and design. For example, if you want higher or more defined cheeks, a stronger jawline, a visible lift, a shaped chin, lighter under-eye circles, remodelled nose, facial shaping or optimization or lines filled.

- On the other hand, skin boosters are for biostimulation to actually reverse time and make your skin younger and deeply hydrated and more supple. It doesn't fill you or solve a specific problem. It simply reduces the early appearance of the signs of ageing.

SKIN CORRECTION

If your goal for your skin is not just maintenance and prevention but the actual treatment of skin issues, don't worry, I have you covered. Here is everything you need to know about corrective skin treatments, related to the specific skin concerns.

Facial hair, body hair and PCOS

For PCOS, I recommend working with your skin doctor, your gynaecologist and an endocrinologist, as needed, for a truly 360-degree care. I always work on the diet and lifestyle of my PCOS clients as I believe PCOS is a lifestyle disease, and also recommend natural supplements as needed. If medications are required, then those are discussed as well in conjunction with the requisite specialists.

For **facial laser hair removal**, I suggest first getting checked for PCOS if you have any of the PCOS symptoms as discussed in chapter 4. That will help determine if you need specialized laser hair removal or customized laser hair removal so that results can be optimized. Most places follow the same one-size-fits-all process for everyone. However, for facial hair, you need to customize the LHR. You want to go to the best centre and spend your hard-earned money, because you want fast results and minimal side effects. You don't want to do thirty sessions. You want it to be done quickly. 'Super hair removal', discussed below, is also an option as it gives faster results, and most technologies are pain-free or nearly painless.

For **body laser hair removal**, go to a centre that is specialized and is dedicated to giving fast results. I have often found that people buy lifetime packages, or cheap laser hair-removal packages of six sessions, and then they have to keep repurchasing. If you have no hormonal condition, 90 per cent of the time, a good laser hair-removal centre should be able to remove 70-90 per cent of a woman's body hair in four to ten sessions. (You need more for men due to their male hormone levels).

Now, if you are the type of person who wants every last hair removed, then laser hair removal will not do that. It maxes out at 70-90 per cent, and does not work on fine hair. If the hair can barely be seen, how can the laser target it? The laser targets the colour in the hair: if it's so thin, or so light-coloured that the human eye can barely register it, then the laser definitely can't get rid of it. Therefore, it obviously also doesn't get rid of white hair. The body also needs a little hair for evolutionary purposes, so it won't allow you to remove 100 per cent of its hair.

Further, as you age and your hormones change, some hair may return, so that's when maintenance sessions are needed. I don't think you should do maintenance sessions willy nilly. Do them only if needed – it means that there is at least 30 per cent hair back on your face or body for you to go for a maintenance session. After all, why should you do a laser maintenance session if there is barely any hair on your skin? It's a bad idea. The laser targets hair: if there is barely any hair, it doesn't work and just becomes a waste of time. I have many patients who haven't needed a maintenance session for years (I am one of them, by the way).

Also, when choosing a laser hair removal session, consider the machines for face or body laser hair removal. Super Hair

Removal is the latest technology out there: it has two or three technologies combined in one machine so the hair is targeted in multiple different ways. So lasers, such as Primelase, Alma Soprano Platinum or Titanium, are good options and combine three different laser wavelengths together. It improves results tremendously, and there are many pain-free options out there too. I also like centres that have two different types of machines because if, for some reason, one machine isn't working on a client, then there is another type for severely resistant hair, so that no one walks out without results. That one, for resistant hair, should typically be a long-pulse Nd:YAG or a microsecond Nd:YAG. But it can even be an alexandrite or diode. IPL (Intense Pulsed Light) is never a good way to get laser hair removal done, because it is just broad band light and not targeted towards hair follicles. It has many different applications, but it is not specialized for hair removal, hence the results are subtle and it requires more sessions than 'super hair removal'.

Risks of laser hair removal

Though a common and safe procedure, which many women safely go through, sometimes, laser hair removal can go awry. Read on for such cases.

Paradoxical hypertrichosis – This is where the hair growth increases instead of decreasing in the area treated. No one knows why this happens, but it's most likely because the energy is too low to kill the hair, so it stimulates it instead. This happens a lot more in patients with PCOS or other hormonal issues, because the hair is already being stimulated by excess hormones, so to destroy the root, it takes a lot more energy than it does for an average person.

Not to worry, it's easy to fix. Just go to a centre with high powered machines and specialized techniques to treat tough hair growth. Ask them if they know how to treat this condition – if they do, try a session or two and see their results. If it's good, go ahead and get rid of that hair!

Burn – Typically, this is rare, but sometimes scabs occur, especially when you have to push energies to treat difficult areas, or when you're treating areas where it's tough to put the handpiece flat on the skin, and finally, also due to simple human error. Get a patch test first to test energies and get comfortable with your centre. If you still end up with a scab or burn, don't worry and tell your practitioner. Typically, they go away within seven days and almost never leave marks.

Pigmentation – I have never seen this happen, to be honest, but I stress on applying sunblock over and over to my clients. Laser hair removal will make you more sensitive to the sun, so tanning can occur if you aren't careful, but it, typically, won't cause pigmentation per se.

Acne – About 6 per cent of laser hair removal results in acne, so get proper post-treatment care and preventative creams to avoid the same.

DR K'S PRO-TIP

Do you have chicken skin or keratosis pilaris? It occurs when keratin gets stuck in the hair follicles and prevents the hair from growing out, resulting in bumps, rashes, little pustules, infections and, sometimes, marks. The more you wax or shave, the more this happens, but it can even happen without waxing or shaving. Many people will report that it occurred suddenly after a waxing session (that's what happened to me). To make this go away, laser hair removal is a must. If there is no hair to grow back, nothing can get stuck under the skin, right? Creams containing AHAs and retinols prevent keratin buildup while also improving the appearance of marks. And for the leftover marks, peels and combination microdermabrasion work well.

Skin correction for acne and rosacea

For acne, I love peels – a succession of proper peels can give great results. They should be done every ten days to two weeks. I combine it with HydraFacial and even some lasers such as NEO and PHOTO HD to reduce inflammation, kill acne and treat those stubborn marks simultaneously.

CLEARSKIN PRO or ERASE-X LASER can be used to reduce oil secretion and kill active zits while gently improving pores and scars.

For rosacea, if there are pimples associated with it or if there is both acne and rosacea, certain gentle peels can be used.

In such cases, PHOTO HD or photofacials are great, and can help with flushing, sensitivity, and redness while also giving the skin a glow. Typically, it requires a different method of treatment with the machine than for acne, but your practitioner will know how to do that. In rosacea, the skin has very reactive blood vessels, with insufficient collagen and elastic tissue, so the vessels have room to dilate a lot causing flushing and breakage in them.[58] So, the more collagen you pack, the less room the vessels have to react. That's why we use PhotoHD (an advanced type of IPL) or lasers or microneedling, to pack in more and more collagen, making the blood vessels less reactive because they don't have the space to go wild.

PEELS

Peels are common everywhere in India, and there are many different kinds out there. Peels need proper sun protection afterwards, and also good post-treatment care to prevent side effects. Go to a proper practitioner who can guide you and tell you which peel will suit your skin and how many sessions you need to take.

For **acne**, peels such as Jessner's peels, TCA peels, mandelic acid and salicylic acid peels will typically purge out zits from under the skin until it's all gone, while also exfoliating dead skin and brightening it as well.

If you have sensitive skin or **rosacea**, then peels with azelaic acid can be beneficial for you. Peels will also work on **pigmentation**, but these take time. Typical ingredients include glycolic acid, although gentler peels may have ingredients such as lactic acid or polyhydroxy acids as well, albeit with lower results.

For anti-ageing, the Yellow Peel or retinol peels can be helpful. The downtime of peels is five to seven days after the procedure, during which there is peeling, dryness and sensitivity to products and sun. Some peels are gentler and have minimal downtime. They can be combined with other treatments as well for better results.

Gold Plasma

If you want that #NoFilter selfie and dewy, supple skin or a red-carpet-worthy skin makeover, this is the treatment for you. This combination treatment is inspired by what Kim Kardashian West swears by before her red carpet appearances, the AquaGold facial. Gold Plasma first exfoliates the skin with mild microdermabrasion, then uses vacuum micro-needling to pull up the skin for perfect contact and, then creates small channels in the skin. A customized combination of baby Botox, PRP, hyaluronic acid and peptides and more, as needed, depending on your concern, are then passed through these channels to stimulate skin cell renewal and boost collagen production. Then an LED boost is given to improve results, followed by an insanely magical gold infusion.

A liquid gold mist is sprayed with oxygen to infuse brightening actives that are mixed with 24k gold for an extra glow boost. The treatment sees a drastic reduction in the signs of ageing, pigmentation, pore size, sebum production, rosacea and acne.

It's great for those who suffer from sensitive skin and rosacea and need a long-lasting glow. Now, we can all keep up with the Kardashians!

Pores

For pores, I recommend microneedling (which we just talked about under 'Prevention'). I also suggest some ablative lasers such as Pixel Perfect or non-ablative lasers such as CLEARSKIN PRO or ERASE-X to boost enough collagen and add to the tightening of pores. Remember, since your pores will dilate, you will need to maintain the results.

In Your City

Look for microneedling with a mixture of baby botox, PRP and actives. It's the mix of PRP and baby botox that helps give glow, hydration and pore reduction.

Pixel perfect

If you need to reduce the appearance of large pores, Pixel Perfect is a laser treatment you can try. It uses a technology called Er:YAG and helps resurface the skin, helping to treat large pores, deep scars, stretch marks or wrinkles. It uses light that goes deep into the skin surface, stimulates the formation of new skin and gets rid of damaged skin cells. Pixel Perfect is also approved by the FDA in the US as one of the most forward, strongest and safest laser methods in fighting deeper skin issues, such as scars and large pores, without the side effects.

You need to know: Numbing cream is usually applied on the treatment area. The duration of the treatment is about thirty minutes for a medium-sized area, and a minimum of six sessions are required for effective results.

There are some after-effects: You will have redness for two days, and tiny scab formation for seven to ten days that will be barely noticeable. But, you should allow two weeks of downtime for everything to get back to normal.

> **In Your City**
>
> Look for ablative Lasers such as CO_2 or Er:YAG that are US FDA-approved; Pixel Perfect is one of those. These should be performed every one to three months, no sooner, and you should go to someone who does these regularly and can boast good results.

Acne scars (and other atrophic scars)

There are lots of types of acne scars, from square boxcars to pitted ice-pick scars to rolling grooves in the skin to even little papular bumps. All are treatable, with the ice pick and papular scars being the hardest to get rid of. The straight truth is that no one can get rid of acne scars 100 per cent, but a lot of scars can be improved with good treatments and a good combination of therapies. And you have to really be patient with it because it does take time! And not all technologies work on all scars – so if one technology isn't working for you, then you may have to shift to another. My favourite is ablative laser resurfacing such as Pixel Perfect (which we just talked about) or CO_2 Laser. I love to combine them with microneedling as well as PRP and the results are phenomenal! But do ensure you go to someone experienced to do this. Only experienced doctors understand how to combine these therapies together and how to best use the technologies to optimize results.

By the way, skin boosters and fillers can be used for last touches on any bigger or stubborn scars that are left post the scar treatment with lasers and microneedling. This is because laser resurfacing and microneedling are more permanent, while filling in scars is less permanent. I have found that if I keep working on scars, they keep getting better, although, after a certain number of sessions, the results are slower. Also, with the technique I use of combining subcision (breaking adhesions under the skin) with filler for filling up stubborn acne scars, the results can last many years there too.

Some brides and grooms even ask me to first fill their scars if they have limited time before an event, and then later come back for laser and microneedling treatment post their event, because filling the scars can be so effective, and it only takes one or two sessions to do.

Acne scars are hard to treat, and usually 60-80 per cent of the results can definitely be achieved. It's the last 20 per cent that takes the longest. So, be patient. They take time, but they are fixable. And quick tip, for that last 20 per cent, consider microneedling facials – you can improve your skin and prevent a lot of the signs of ageing; at the same time, ask your doc to work on the scars – so your regular sessions become not only treating the scars, but also a preventative measure!

Stretch marks (Striae)

Stretch marks can be either purplish-red or white. Typically, they occur because the skin stretches beyond its elastic capability, so it essentially breaks in the lower levels, causing those tiger stripes. When they are new, they are red or purple because they are fresh. At this time they are the easiest to treat. Nearly 60-90 per cent can be removed with technologies such as ablative lasers like CO_2 Laser and Pixel Perfect, and even deep microneedling of depths more than 1.0 mm, if treated at this time. These lasers have a downtime of seven to ten days during which your skin can have little bumps and can feel stingy for a day or two. But boy do they work, and the side effects are negligible. For the colour of the striae, we can even use Q-switched lasers or lasers like CLEARLIFT 4D, which is a fractionated Q-switched laser, and if you don't want any downtime, then CLEARSKIN PRO or FRAXEL Lasers using an Er: Glass technology can help too.

Now, once the striae are white and old, they become harder to treat. Microneedling can be used in addition to ablative lasers, but the results end up at 50-60 per cent. But the texture really improves, so it's still worth it. Combining the two technologies together can give you some amazing results.

DR K'S PRO-TIP

Fancy creams to treat your stretch marks? Don't waste
your time. They typically take advantage of the natural
process of stretch marks turning from purple to white, so
you feel like the fancy expensive oil magically improved
your stretch marks. Instead, work on improving your
skin's elasticity to prevent stretch marks by applying
cocoa butter, coconut oil, and even a retinol lotion if you
don't have sun exposure.

Pigmentation

Essentially, when treating pigmentation, your practitioner will
diagnose the pigmentation disease, how deep the discolouration
is, and get a history of what caused it. If it's some simple red-
coloured marks, then photofacials or Intense Pulsed Light
can be really effective. But if there are darker marks or patches
or whole areas that are brown to grey-black in colour, then
we look at different options. Here, we consider peels based
on your lifestyle and how much time you have, as peels can
take numerous sessions to show effects. We also love to
add microneedling, because it delivers anti-pigmentation
actives into the deeper layers of the skin, while also training
keratinocytes how to behave better over time, so the next time
they get exposed to trauma, they don't react so badly and cause
as much pigmentation. Skin specialists love microneedling for
that purpose: it is effective, as well as preventive as a solution.

Finally, we get to the good stuff – LASERS! I love lasers, and I'm American Board Certified in them, so that is literally my wheelhouse. Lasers such as Q-switched Nd:YAG lasers have definitely been the go-to for most pigmentation issues, but each laser is different and works differently, even if they all are Q-switched Nd:YAG. Excitingly, lasers such as PICOSURE have changed the game at getting rid of tough pigmentation with fewer sessions. It can also improve your complexion. I would definitely recommend Picosure or Pico-based lasers for tough-to-treat pigmentation and if you want fast results. Besides the laser type, the efficacy of your results will also depend on who your laser practitioner is: it is important how they use their machine and how much experience they have.

Melasma, however, is a special case, where we treat inside out and have to proceed slowly and gently: with microneedling and gentle lasers. This is because melasma is triggered not only by the sun but also by your hormones. So stress, hormonal variation, and irritation can actually worsen the situation. It's important to treat it gently, and then once it's better, maintenance will be required.

Dullness

Dullness or complexion issues are common concerns, and diet and skincare can definitely help in this, as discussed in our previous chapters. While therapies help too, no treatment can remove your dullness entirely, without you also doing your part of dietary changes, sleep, stress reduction, exercise, water consumption and proper skincare. So, before you start berating your dermatologist, remember that you also have to work on it. Now, when our skin is exposed to trauma, or sun, or even major illnesses, melanin gets released into it, causing some tanning. This melanin release is a sign of skin damage, and the melanin is made and deposited to prevent further damage.

How to treat this? Easy ways to treat this include, therapies such as microdermabrasion, where we use either crystals or stones, such as diamonds, to exfoliate off the superficial layer of the skin, thereby, getting rid of the damaged skin layer. (Caution: avoid this if you have sensitive or rosacea-prone skin, or if you have a lot of comedones). Peels, which are discussed in the acne section, are also used to treat this. Glow peels with polyhydroxy acids or lactic acid or even vitamin C peels can be very helpful in getting rid of dull and dead/tanned/damaged skin. I like to combine microdermabrasion with a custom brightening serum, followed by LED light for dullness and tan removal in my facial BRIGHT LIGHTS at my clinic.

AGEING

I know we talked about preventing ageing earlier. But what if you are already seeing signs of ageing? Can you get those corrected? The answer is: a 100 per cent yes!

So how do you know if you need treatment for ageing? What are the signs? Lines and wrinkles, textural irregularities and sagging. Below is a note on everything you need to know about lines and wrinkles, followed by sagging. You will see that most of the treatments work for all these indications, but I have split it up, so you can see where each one fits in. Remember, the skin has three layers and ageing hits all three. The wrinkles and sagging segment typically discusses the lower half of the second layer to the third layer of the skin, but the rest of the issues, such as enlarged pores, poor texture, age spots, discolouration and more, still need to be dealt with. For complete skin rejuvenation, include all three layers! So remember, for textural issues, pores and more superficial lines that are static or non-dynamic, Laser resurfacing with Pixel Perfect, or Non-ablative lasers such as CLEARLIFT 4D and CLEARSKIN PRO, will still be needed. Microneedling can also be considered here, but it should be customized for your skin issues such as depth of pores, lines, or severity of discolouration and textural irregularity.

Wrinkles 101: Everything you need to know

What causes wrinkles?

One of the most prominent causes of early wrinkles is exposure to UV rays. Sun damage can show up in the form of early wrinkling of the skin. Another cause of wrinkles is dehydrated skin, along with the frequent consumption of alcohol and smoking. Wrinkles can start off as fine lines and then go on to develop into deep-set folds. Initially, many wrinkles are dynamic, so they only happen when you use the muscle, for example, when you frown. But as time goes on, those grooves stay and become static. The beginning of wrinkles can happen as early as at the age of twenty-five, which is why it is recommended that you start with a micro-ageing skincare routine once you hit the second half of your twenties.

How to prevent wrinkles

The best way to prevent wrinkles from showing up earlier than they should is to follow a regular skincare routine that promotes skin cell turnover and keeps your skin hydrated and moisturized. Wearing enough sunscreen and reapplying it every time you're out in the sun can also help prevent wrinkles caused by UV damage. And, of course, the lesser your alcohol consumption and smoking frequency, the better it is for your skin.

How effective are non-surgical anti-ageing treatments for wrinkles?

Non-surgical anti-ageing treatments can be extremely effective in treating the areas of your skin that have started to wrinkle as well as in promoting healthy, younger skin. You don't always need to sign up for intensive surgery or go under the knife to achieve better, more youthful skin. Non-surgical treatments are available in a wide range going from facials to fillers and even PRP: you're sure to find one that fits your needs perfectly.

Benefits of non-invasive anti-ageing treatments

The benefits of non-invasive anti-ageing treatments are plenty, making them a popular choice to tackle signs of ageing:

- The treatments are non-invasive, thus, drastically reducing downtime.

- Since they're not permanent, they can be altered to meet your skin's current requirements each time you go for your next session.

- In case of a skin reaction, it can be easily controlled and treated due to the treatment's non-invasive nature.

INJECTABLES

PRP and skin boosters

PRP and skin boosters can be used to fill wrinkles, do some mild lifting as well as prevent ageing, but it has already been discussed before, so let's move on to the fun stuff!

Botox

Botox is unarguably one of the most popular treatments for wrinkles because of its efficacy and targeted nature. Botox is short for Botulinum Toxin A, which is a protein that gently paralyses muscles in the area where it is injected, preventing creasing and folding, a.k.a wrinkles. There are many brands of Botulinum Toxin out there, but let's simply call it all Botox, which is a brand of Juvederm. If you're dealing with dynamic wrinkling and creasing around your forehead, the eye area and the mouth, this treatment can make your face look years younger and smoothen wrinkles easily.

> **DR K'S PRO-TIP**
>
> Dynamic wrinkles are those that happen only when you use the muscles, like when you frown or smile. Botox doesn't work so much on static lines that are there no matter what you do – for those, laser resurfacing or non-ablative lasers and microneedling are better. But typically, you will need both Botox to prevent dynamic wrinkling and treatments to reduce static wrinkles in order to prevent further lines from forming or to prevent existing lines from getting worse.

Botox also helps tighten the neck and jawline. I have even used it to remove a gummy smile and reduce wrinkles around the mouth and on the chin. For aesthetic purposes, Botox can be used to lengthen your chin, narrow your jawline by injecting the masseters, narrow your nostrils, lift the tip of the nose, and give your lips a lift. Botox, in the hands of an expert, can make you look naturally younger and optimize your features.

Fillers

The idea behind fillers is to get it right. So how to get it right? Look to improve the lines and folds, but not to get rid of them entirely. Perfection makes you look like a strange ageless cyborg. Aiming to look like yourself is important. And build up slowly. Remember, too much, and you get a pillow face. Here is everything you need to know about dermal fillers.

Dermal Fillers 101: Everything you should know about fillers

What are dermal fillers?

Dermal fillers make use of hyaluronic acid – a naturally occurring substance in our skin – to lift and plump skin. While you can get fillers for your entire face, they can also be injected to lift and reshape certain areas of your face like the jaw and the chin. The natural fillers are injected in small controlled doses just under the surface of the skin to fill out sunken areas and lines, boost collagen production and give a smoother, firmer and more refreshed appearance. They're a popular anti-ageing treatment of choice due to their low-maintenance nature and natural-looking results.

Dermal fillers are made of gel-like substances, the most popular choice being hyaluronic acid. Hyaluronic acid naturally occurs in our body as well, giving us a plump and hydrated look. Over the years, as we age, our bodies start to produce less of this acid and that starts to show in the form of signs of ageing such as dehydration, sagging skin, fine lines and wrinkles. This is why, when you religiously apply hyaluronic acid topically or get a dermal filler, your skin starts to look younger and more nourished.

There's barely any downtime associated with the treatment and the fact that the results aren't permanent allows you to experiment with just how much you need. The trick is to go about it in a gently transformative way to maintain a natural look. No one should be able to tell that you have had fillers, unless you want them to know.

Which dermal fillers do I need?

Fillers may sound intimidating, but there's no reason to fret. I am here to ease your worries. There are three main filler brands – Juvederm, Boletero and Restylane – and each of them has different subtypes. These are completely natural and made of hyaluronic acid. Each filler subtype has different rheological properties that I won't go into here, but your experienced practitioner will know which filler, which brand and which type to use for your needs.

Which areas can dermal fillers treat?

Dermal fillers can be used for the basics like laugh lines, marionette lines, forehead lines, temple hollowing, facelifting, under-eye hollows, and lip fillers. But there are also other aesthetic purposes to use fillers, such as jawline enhancement for men and women, facial balancing, forehead shaping and filling, chin augmentation, creating chin dimples, chin lengthening and smoothening, cheek filling, lip designing, non-invasive nose jobs, facial proportion balancing, line reduction, injectable highlighting of favourite areas such as your cheekbones, nose reshaping, brow lifts and more. There is profile balancing as well, which is facial optimization with gentle tweaks to softly enhance your features. Besides this, fillers are also used for neck, hand and feet rejuvenation, breast and butt augmentation and lifting, and cellulite improvement for areas other than the face.

Under-eyes and **lips** are the most common places where people get fillers. The under eye is a popular area for fillers because it's safe, and the hollow goes away just like that! Lip augmentation is also common, because no lip plumper will give you the lips you have been dreaming of. I like to do a natural lip lift technique, where I work with your lip architecture to build better lips that look like yours, without the trout pout. Natural lip effects are easy to achieve in the hands of an experienced practitioner, and you should find one who has done this and understands your vision, while also guiding you on what won't work for you.

What can you expect during your treatment?

Getting a dermal filler may sound daunting, but it's a fairly straightforward and painless process. Once you and your aesthetic doctor have decided on the exact points that need to be injected, a comprehensive plan is created for the procedure. Numbing cream is applied if required, and then your skin is injected with the filler in small doses and gently massaged in place. The entire procedure takes between thirty to forty minutes, and the results can also be micro-reversed on request so that they can be titrated perfectly.

How long do the results last?

The longevity of your dermal fillers depends on the exact filler used, the area it's been injected in, and your metabolism. They can last anywhere between six to twenty-four months or even more. If you'd specifically like to have the kind that lasts the longest, make sure you discuss that with your doctor in advance.

Do dermal fillers have any side effects?

Dermal fillers are made of natural hyaluronic acid that is safely injected into your skin. Side effects associated with it are rare. There is a small risk that the filler can enter a blood vessel, and rare cases of blindness and stroke have been reported. That being said, tens of millions of fillers are performed around the world, and these side effects are very rare, few and far between. Usually, it's very safe as long as all precautions are followed. You may usually only experience slight redness, bruising or swelling for up to a week, which is the duration of recovery, after your treatment is done.

What does recovery look like?

Dermal fillers do not have weeks of downtime associated with them, making them the perfect treatment to get, even during your lunchtime break. As I mentioned, there may be some redness, bruising or mild swelling for three to seven days. If you're not 100 per cent happy with your results post recovery, the procedure can be reversed or altered to give you the desired result.

In Your City

Look for a practitioner who has carried out thousands of filler and Botox procedures, so they know how to make it look natural and can work with the movement of your face so you look like yourself, only younger. I believe in facial optimization and tiny tweaks to gently change your appearance and keep you looking younger, without making you look artificial. I will often say no when you want perfection or all your lines filled or 100 per cent symmetry, because that, typically, will look fake. A real face has some gentle lines and a little asymmetry. Look for a practitioner who understands your aesthetic and who can bring your vision to life.

Sagging

What is sagging? Sagging is when gravity takes a toll on your skin. Over time, you find your face drooping, your jowls become prominent, your jawline becomes weaker, your under-eye hollows get deeper, your lips look thinner and even your nose droops. Your neck will also bear the signs of sagging – turkey neck, the term for that dreaded neck sag, is a rather hated word. A face that was shaped like an upside-down triangle, will now look more square due to all that drooping.

Why does sagging happen? Over time, fat reduces, the skin loses laxity and elasticity, and even the bones end up resorbing, so that the skin just hangs down more.

We can treat sagging invasively and non-invasively. We have already discussed non-invasive treatments with Ulthera and non-invasive facelifting technologies in the anti-ageing segment. Invasive treatments for sagging include Botox and fillers (which we have just talked about), and thread lifts.

THREAD LIFT 101

What is a thread lift?

A thread lift is a skin firming and lifting anti-ageing facial treatment that targets the skin around your chin, jawline and neck area. We make use of thin, absorbable threads to induce collagen production in the areas that need it the most, making your face appear sharper and more lifted.

The thread lift treatment involves implanting fine, absorbable threads (such as the ones we use when we get stitches) into the subcutaneous layer of the skin to induce collagen stimulation. There are different types of threads available, from basic PDO threads to COG threads to suspension threads and more. Trust your practitioner on what threads they feel will suit your concern best. Threads are pretty comfortable and feel just like acupuncture, and are a quick and easy way to induce collagen production and tightening. Newer thread procedures are safe, come with low risk, and take all of fifteen to twenty minutes to do after which you can resume a normal life.

What are the advantages of a thread lift in comparison to a facelift?

A thread lift requires no surgery, lasers, injections or upkeep! On the other hand, a facelift is an invasive surgery, and the risk of complications are much higher than those in a thread lift. If you're not satisfied with the results of your thread lift, they can be tweaked to suit what you want. If you do get a facelift, however, you will need to sign up for another invasive treatment to make alterations. A thread lift is also easier on your pocket than a facelift.

There is also **non-surgical face tightening**, which involves the usage of technologies that painlessly heat deeper layers of your skin to boost collagen production and tighten the skin. These technologies typically use radiofrequency energy (radio waves), near-infrared light or ultrasound as the method for heating the skin, or a combination of them, thereby triggering collagen synthesis. There are also different types: some are gentler and require multiple sessions, while others need one session in a year. If you are getting an Ulthera or Thermage, which is a single-session non-invasive facelift technology that gives long results, then that energy is being delivered more specifically deeper into the skin layers, and a lot more of it, that's why you can get a non-invasive lift with long-lasting results. Now, say you have your results of face tightening but you want more? Then threads can often be added afterwards for extra results in areas where you want extra lifting. Threads are wonderful to add whenever you want an extra face or brow lift, jawline tightening, cheek lifting, neck tightening, and even breast, tummy and butt tightening.

Thread lift vs dermal fillers

While dermal fillers do lift and plump your skin, they are better for filling lines, creases, wrinkles and hollows on your face. A thread lift is a better-suited treatment to look after sagging skin that's lost its elasticity around the jaw and neck, without the extra volume of fillers. It's also a great non-surgical way to get cat-eyes or a brow lift. In fact, it may be of merit to discuss getting both treatments with your aesthetic doctor to get the best of both worlds and a more youthful look overall.

What can you expect after the treatment?

Some redness and mild swelling may occur around the injection site for three to seven days after your treatment, and there may be some tenderness for four to ten days. Very rarely, you may observe some inflammation in the area, and sometimes, the threads can be visible as well, but these can be removed and taken care of at the clinic itself.

How long do the results last?

Results take up to three months to show and last for six months to two years. The practitioner will choose different threads based on your concerns.

Any side effects?

Thread lifts do not come with the risk of severe side effects, since it is a non-invasive treatment with dissolvable threads. You will only experience some mild swelling and redness for a maximum duration of a week or two. Tenderness and a sensation of lumpiness are common for up to two to three weeks, although it is usually unnoticeable. Rarely, you can experience puckering in the area, which requires some gentle massage or, sometimes, a little RF (radiofrequency) in the clinic. In case, you do spot any inflammation or irritation, that can be taken care of easily.

Who should get a thread lift and who should avoid the procedure?

For those of you who want a natural-looking appearance without the volume of fillers, a thread lift is the perfect choice. If you have skin that is heavily sagging, a thread lift may not be the best solution for you. As is the case with skincare, treatments are recommended on a case-to-case basis, after a thorough analysis of your skin during a consultation.

Skin doctors are cool (they are!)

Nowadays, there are so many cool things we skin doctors can do that you never knew, and without any surgeries involved! We can treat your cellulite and stretch marks. That chicken skin, known as keratosis pilaris, or little bumps/marks on the arms, legs, or back – we can get rid of them all with laser hair removal, followed by peels and therapies to remove the remaining marks.

We can even do non-invasive fat loss, tighten your double chin, your neck, your breasts, your butt and your tummy. We can treat your hair loss, and even augment your breasts and butt with fillers and/or PRP. The dry and aged skin on your hands and feet can be improved with fillers, skin boosters, PRP, lasers and peels for a full-on 360-degree rejuvenation. That pesky pigmentation on your back and arms, known as cutaneous macular amyloidosis? Also treatable. Even your knee lines or 'knickles' (as we like to call them) can be blasted away with a little PRP.

One of my favourite things you didn't know that cosmetologists & dermatologists can do? A non-invasive nose job. I say nose job and you think surgery, right? It doesn't have to be.

Everything you should know about getting a non-surgical nose job, i.e., a nose filler

If you're particularly conscious of your nose and you'd like for it to look a certain way – less wide, slightly shorter in length, or smoother overall – it can be done in a minimally invasive. Enter: a non-surgical nose job or rhinoplasty. Plastic surgery often comes with a lot of downtime and can seem daunting to sign up for, especially for first-timers. A non-surgical nose job can help, without you having to worry about surgical intervention, but it's a decision best taken with your dermatologist or aesthetic doctor.

What is a non-surgical nose job?

A non-surgical nose job or a nose filler is an in-clinic procedure, wherein the practitioner will evaluate your current nose, measure it and understand how to reshape it in the best way possible according to your face shape. They make use of liquid fillers to inject areas of your nose that need lifting, to create the perfect nose for your face shape and one that works in tandem with the rest of your features. Threads can also be used to lift your nose or to narrow the width of your nostril flair, and Botox to prevent the tip of the nose from moving downwards when you smile.

How does it work?

When we do a non-surgical rhinoplasty, we look at the bridge of the nose, dorsal humps (the bumps on the nose, also called the nasal bridge), the nasolabial angle and also the angle between the nose and the chin. All of these things allow us to design a great nose with non-surgical options, such as fillers, as opposed to an invasive surgery. With fillers, one can easily improve the angle of the nose bridge. For example, if it's too sharp, it can be made smooth and gentle. If there are any dorsal humps or bumps, we can fill them in. In fact, when something looks less bumpy and more smooth, it also looks less wide. The bumpier it is, the more your eye is attracted to the bump, making it look wider. The options are endless and, more importantly, customized to your specific face and needs. The best part is that whatever you don't like is 100 per cent reversible and can even be tweaked a little, so it doesn't all go to waste.

Which areas are targeted as part of this procedure?

The areas that are targeted for a non-surgical nasal rhinoplasty depend on the requirements for your nose. If we need to lift a drooping nasal tip, we will work only on filling that area to push it upwards like a cartilage graft. This makes your nose appear more aesthetically pleasing without the need for any invasive surgery at all. If you'd like to smoothen the entire nose and get rid of all bumps, we will need to use the filler over the entire length of your nose.

Fillers can also be used to create a makeup-like effect, just like you use a highlighter along the centre of your nose to make it look more narrow. When we use a thin vertical line of the filler down your nose, the filler makes your nose reflect light just like a highlighter does and makes it appear more contoured without you having to use any products. Consider it to be the 'I woke up like this' adage come to life.

If your nose to chin angle is too large, the nose projects forward more than the chin – this can be fixed by projecting the chin instead. We call this the Tinkerbell lift. Adding a filler to your chin, if your nose is too large, makes your nose appear smaller and more proportionate.

Now, I am sure that you are feeling really optimistic knowing how much is available out there to help fix your concerns. But keep in mind that you still need to maintain those results. After all, exposure to pollution, sun, blue light and dirt/dust doesn't just stop. So, let's move on to how you can maintain your skin.

SKIN MAINTENANCE

Once you think you have achieved the skin you love, work towards maintaining it. Just like the rest of our being, our skin also needs some TLC (tender loving care). Some hydration, some cleansing, some love, and your skin can be ready to take on the world! And if this is what you think your skin needs, here are some of my favourite maintenance ritual treatments.

Blackheads

For those of you who are concerned about blackheads, my recommendation is HydraFacial, which can be done monthly. Honestly, I am not a fan of salon facials and cleanups. Did you know 50 per cent of salon facials have been associated with breakouts? I would not recommend that. My favourite HydraFacial is Elixir, which is also available at Isya.

If you are plagued with blackheads and whiteheads and/or have combination skin that needs a glow, HydraFacial, which I call The Elixir, is a good option for you. It starts with lymphatic drainage and is, then, followed by a cleanse and peel that exfoliates skin and sloughs off dead skin cells that clog pores.

Then a painless suction wand helps remove the debris clogging them. A hydrating moisturizer is packed on to lock the moisture and fight dryness, and the skin is loaded with antioxidants and peptides to maximize your glow.

Sometimes, we may also use manual extraction to remove hard to reach blackheads. The result? Reduced acne and oil production with a maximized glow.

You need to know: You can sneak in this sixty-minute ritual in your lunchtime and you'll see immediate results. You can schedule this treatment on a monthly basis for maximum effect.

Nearly no after-effects: Some people may experience a little purging of acne that's under the skin, but this clears in a few days.

In Your City

Look for someone who performs hydrafacial, and doesn't skimp on the ingredients. If the price is too low and too good to be true, it probably is. You want the best, so get the best! Do this monthly.

Beyond the face

It's not just about your face. Don't forget your neck, chest, hands and feet. These are the neglected areas, and they show your real age. A lot of the treatments that we have talked about here can be used to rejuvenate these areas as well.

Don't get overwhelmed

That's a lot to absorb, right? Listen, and go by what you want to get done. You don't have to do everything at once. Focus on each concern and treat those over a period of time. If we are talking about just the face, a good plan and an expert doctor can make your life easy and you don't have to come in more than once a month. And if your skin is really well-maintained and you have completed prevention procedures as needed, then even quarterly visits to the clinic are good enough. The best way to go about it is to discuss with your practitioner what you are looking for and what your time and budget constraints are. They will work with you to find a solution or to create a different timeline, so you can get what you want without all the hassle and stress.

Now, clearly, I have blown your mind with everything that is possible in dermatology and aesthetics. But here is where I caution you. This book is designed to educate and guide you on all of your options. It is up to you what you do with this. Power is a great responsibility, and the power of knowledge is now yours. As I said in the very beginning, you are on a journey of self-discovery and beauty. If you go about it with fear and insecurity, you will often make the wrong choices and end up not feeling happy or secure with your decisions. But, if you come from a place of awareness, self-acceptance and self-love, you will end up making educated choices that will help you get the results you truly want and will feel good about. Because that's the real goal, right? To feel good, in the here and now, and within your own skin.

GLOSSARY

- Acanthosis nigricans: Dark, velvety hyperpigmentation in areas like the back of the neck, underarms, knuckles or groin.

- AHA: Alpha hydroxy acids are small to large acids that stimulate exfoliation of skin cells and are often used in pigmentation, hydration, and glow. They include ingredients like glycolic acid, lactic acid, and malic acid.

- Alopecia: A symptom showing hair loss or patches of hair loss. There are many diseases that cause alopecia, such as alopecia areata.

- BHA: Beta hydroxy acids are oil soluble, and can remove sebum, and unobstruct pores – salicylic acid is an example.

- Botox: A brand of botulinum toxin that is designed to relax muscles.

- Clean beauty: A marketing term designed to make you believe a product is all natural; but has no basis in actual federal legislation regarding cosmetic products.

- Cutaneous macular amyloidosis: A common skin condition where a harmless protein gets deposited into the skin, causing the appearance of hyperpigmented patches. Typically happens on the back and arms.

- Dermabrasion or microdermabrasion: Removing the top layers of skin using abrasive tools like diamond tips or aluminium oxide crystals.

- Fillers: An injectable that is used to fill up lines and hollows, lift and contour. Usually, it is made of Hyaluronic acid.

- Hirsutism: Excess hair growth on women in a male distribution pattern. For example, a beard, neck hair, chest hair, tummy hair, thigh hair and more.

- Hyaluronic acid: A sugar that is naturally present in the skin. It is a skincare active that is a humectant, so it helps boost the hydration in skin. It is also the primary ingredient in HA based fillers and in skin boosters.

- Hyperandrogenism: A condition where there is an excess circulation of male hormones. This can result in acne, balding and excess hair growth on the body and face.

- Insulin resistance: Where your body makes more and more insulin to absorb the glucose your body breaks food down into.

- Keratinocytes: The primary type of cell present in the topmost layer of the skin, the epidermis.

- Laser hair removal: A process where a machine uses a concentrated beam of light to target and kill hair, resulting in overall hair reduction.

- LED masks: A home device that uses low level light therapy to boost collagen, reduce acne and soothe the skin.

- Malar areas: The bilateral cheek areas right next to the nose.

- Melasma: A type of pigmentation that is often associated with pregnancy or hormonal changes that makes you more sensitive to the sun.

- Micro needling: The use of multiple microns-sized fine needles to help improve the skin, boost collagen, and infuse ingredients into the skin.

- Moisture sandwich: A method to increase moisturization of the skin through the application of a mist, a serum with a strong humectant like hyaluronic acid on top of the mist to bind the water, and then a moisturizer with an emollient to hold the moisture in the skin.

- Ochronosis: A bluish-black discolouration of the skin that can happen from certain metabolic diseases, but rarely can occur due to topical actives like hydroquinone, resorcinol, or benzene.

- PCOS: Polycystic Ovarian Syndrome is a syndrome that affects women of reproductive age that can result in irregular periods, infertility, multiple cysts in ovaries, and excess male hormone (androgen) secretion.

- Peptides: Peptides are anti-ageing ingredients, typically messenger molecules that stimulate fibroblasts to increase collagen and elastin secretion.

- PHA: Polyhydroxy acid is considered the second generation of the Alpha hydroxy acid, which is gentler and less sensitizing than AHAs. The molecules are bigger and are effective at hydration and increasing glow and cell turnover. Examples include, gluconolactone and lactobionic acid.

- Pigmentation: The appearance of darker appearing skin. It can occur due to a variety of diseases, trauma, products and conditions. It is a symptom, not a disease.
- PRP: Platelet-rich plasma derived from one's own blood to stimulate rejuvenation and healing.
- Retinol: A type of Retinoid which is derived from Vitamin A and is known to boost collagen and elastin.
- Rhinoplasty: A nose job.
- Seborrheic dermatitis: A type of harmless rash that looks red, greasy with mild scale. It can occur on the face, chest, back and scalp. It is the most common cause of dandruff.
- UVA: A type of ultraviolet light emitted by the sun, which is associated with skin ageing and pigmentation. It is also associated with skin cancer.
- UVB: A type of ultraviolet light emitted by the sun, which is known to cause tanning and skin burn. It is also associated with skin cancer.

NOTES

1. Yin Z. Hessefort, Brian T. Holland, and Richard W. Cloud, 'True porosity measurement of hair: A new way to study hair damage mechanisms', *J. Cosmet Sci.* 59 (July/August, 2008): 303–15, http://beauty-review.nl/wp-content/uploads/2014/06/True-porosity-measurement-of-hair-A-new-way-to-study-hair-damage-mechanisms.pdf

2. Maria Fernanda Reis Gavazzoni Dias, Andréia Munck de Almeida, Patricia Makino Rezende Cecato, Andre Ricardo Adriano, and Janine Pichler, 'The Shampoo pH can Affect the Hair: Myth or Reality?' *International Journal of Trichology* Vol. 6, no. 3 (July-September 2014): 95–99, doi:10.4103/0974-7753.139078, https://www.ncbi.nlm.nih.gov/pmc/articles/PMC4158629/

3. https://scholar.google.com/scholar?hl=en&as_sdt=0%2C5&q=hair+frizz&btnG=

4. Aarti S. Rele and R. B. Mohile, 'Effect of mineral oil, sunflower oil, and coconut oil on prevention of hair damage', *J. Cosmet Sci.* 54; (March/April 2003): 175–92, http://beauty-review.nl/wp-content/uploads/2014/06/Effect-of-mineral-oil-sunflower-oil-and-coconut-oil-on-prevention-of-hair-damage.pdf

5. http://science-yhairblog.blogspot.com/2013/06/oils-which-ones-soak-in-vs-coat-hair.html

6. Erling Thom, 'Stress and the Hair Growth Cycle: Cortisol-Induced Hair Growth Disruption', *Journal of Drugs in Dermatology* Vol. 15, no. 8; (August 2016), https://jddonline.com/articles/dermatology/S1545961616P1001X/2

7. http://beauty-review.nl/wp-content/uploads/2014/06/True-porosity-measurement-of-hair-A-new-way-to-study-hair-damage-mechanisms.pdf

8. https://www.aad.org/public/everyday-care/nail-care-secrets/basics/pedicures/reduce-artificial-nail-damage

9. https://www.aad.org/public/everyday-care/nail-care-secrets/basics/pedicures/gel-manicures

10. https://www.ijdvl.com/article.asp?issn=0378-6323%3Byear%3D2007%3Bvolume%3D73%3Bissue%3D1%3Bspage%3D22%3Bepage%3D25%3Baulast%3DEnshaieh;source=post_page----

11. https://onlinelibrary.wiley.com/doi/pdf/10.1111/ajd.12465

12. http://v2.practicaldermatology.com/pdfs/PD0905%20CosChallenge.pdf

13. http://www.grimalt.net/wp-content/uploads/2013/04/parabens-2013.pdf

14. Federica Guardo, Maria Cerana, Gisella D'urso, Fortunato Genovese, and Marco Palumbo, 'Male PCOS equivalent and nutritional restriction: Are we stepping forward?' *Medical Hypotheses* (2019), 126. 10.1016/j.mehy.2019.03.003

15. https://www.nhs.uk/conditions/polycystic-ovary-syndrome-pcos/diagnosis/

16. https://www.ncbi.nlm.nih.gov/pmc/articles/PMC4161081/pdf/jcs-1-183.pdf

17. https://www.aafp.org/afp/2016/0715/p106.html
18. https://www.aafp.org/afp/2016/0715/p106.html
19. A.J. Duleba and A. Dokras, 'Is PCOS an inflammatory process?' *Fertil Steril* 97, no. 1 (2012): 7–12, doi:10.1016/j.fertnstert.2011.11.023
20. B.O. Yildiz and R. Azziz, 'The adrenal and polycystic ovary syndrome,' *Rev Endocr Metab Disord* 8 (2007): 331–42, https://doi.org/10.1007/s11154-007-9054-0
21. Carlos Moran, Ricardo Azziz, 'The Role Of The Adrenal Cortex In Polycystic Ovary Syndrome,' *Obstetrics and Gynecology Clinics of North America* 28, no. 1 (2001): 63–75, ISSN 0889-8545
22. https://adaa.org/understanding-anxiety/related-illnesses/other-related-conditions/stress/physical-activity-reduces-st
23. https://www.ncbi.nlm.nih.gov/pmc/articles/PMC3894304/
24. https://systematicreviewsjournal.biomedcentral.com/articles/10.1186/s13643-019-0962-3
25. https://academic.oup.com/humrep/article/23/3/642/2914018
26. https://www.researchgate.net/profile/Brenda_Bruner/publication/6887428_Effects_of_exercise_and_nutritional_counseling_in_women_with_polycystic_ovary_syndrome/links/56bcf6e908aed69599460b47/Effects-of-exercise-and-nutritional-counseling-in-women-with-polycystic-ovary-syndrome.pdf
27. https://www.aafp.org/afp/2012/0801/p244.html#:~:text=Data%20derived%20from%20the%20National,in%20females%20than%20in%20males
28. https://www.cdc.gov/diabetes/basics/diabetes.html
29. https://dermnetnz.org/topics/skin-problems-associated-with-diabetes-mellitus
30. https://www.scientificamerican.com/article/soil-depletion-and-nutrition-loss/

31. https://www.sciencedirect.com/science/article/abs/pii/S0013935114004563

32. https://www.businessinsider.in/slideshows/miscellaneous/9-terrifying-things-that-could-be-lurking-in-your-tap-water/slidelist/68838985.cms#slideid=68838993

33. https://www.jagranjosh.com/general-knowledge/what-types-of-toxins-are-present-in-tap-water-1531484527-1

34. https://www.nrdc.org/stories/whats-your-drinking-water

35. https://www.scientificamerican.com/article/soil-depletion-and-nutrition-loss/

36. https://www.aad.org/public/diseases/a-z/diabetes-warning-signs

37. https://www.tandfonline.com/doi/pdf/10.4161/derm.22028

38. https://www.tandfonline.com/doi/pdf/10.4161/derm.22028

39. K. Michaelson, A. Wolk, S. Langenskiöld, S. Basu, E. Warensjö Lemming, H. Melhus et al. Milk intake and risk of mortality and fractures in women and men: cohort studies *BMJ* 2014; 349 :g6015 doi:10.1136/bmj.g6015

40. C.A. Adebamowo, D. Spiegelman, et al., 'High school dietary dairy intake and teenage acne,' *J Am Acad Dermatol* 52, no. 2 (2005): 2075–14

41. K. Michaelson, A. Wolk, S. Langenskiöld, S. Basu, E. Warensjö Lemming, H. Melhus et al. Milk intake and risk of mortality and fractures in women and men: cohort studies *BMJ* 2014; 349 :g6015 doi:10.1136/bmj.g6015

42. M.M. Kober and W.P. Bowe, 'The effect of probiotics on immune regulation, acne, and photoaging,' *Int J Womens Dermatol* 1, no. 2 (2015): 85–89, doi:10.1016/j. ijwd.2015.02.001

43. https://www.vegrecipesofindia.com/how-to-make-almond-milk/

44. https://sharan-india.org/recipes/oats-milk/

45. https://www.vegrecipesofindia.com/how-to-make-coconut-milk/#wprm-recipe-container-137892

46. https://gut.bmj.com/content/gutjnl/68/8/1516.full.pdf

47. https://gut.bmj.com/content/gutjnl/68/8/1516.full.pdf

48. https://www.hsph.harvard.edu/nutritionsource/antioxidants/

49. https://www.webmd.com/diet/features/antioxidant-superstars-vegetables-and-beans#1

50. https://www.webmd.com/food-recipes/news/20040617/antioxidants-found-unexpected-foods#:~:text=Researchers%20found%20that%20small%20red,rich%20foods%20studied%20were%20beans.

51. https://www.ncbi.nlm.nih.gov/pmc/articles/PMC3257681/

52. https://www.hsph.harvard.edu/nutritionsource/healthy-eating-plate-vs-usda-myplate/

53.

54. https://www.ncbi.nlm.nih.gov/pmc/articles/PMC3667300/

55. N. Arjmandi, G. Mortazavi, S. Zarei, M. Faraz, S.A.R. Mortazavi, 'Can Light Emitted from Smartphone Screens and Taking Selfies Cause Premature Aging and Wrinkles?' *J Biomed Phys Eng.* 8, no. 4 (2018): 447–52

56. C. Chamayou-Robert, C. DiGiorgio, O. Brack, O. Doucet, 'Blue light induces DNA damage in normal human skin keratinocytes. Photodermatol Photoimmunol Photomed,' 15 July 2021, doi: 10.1111/phpp.12718 (Epub ahead of print. PMID: 34265135)

57. https://www.profhilo.co.in/

58. John Jesitus, 'Collagen Degeneration Linked to Rosacea', *Dermatology Times* 42, no. 4 (April 2021).

59. https://www.dermatologytimes.com/view/collagen-degeneration-linked-to-rosacea

Additional Notes:

1. http://www.isyaderm.com/pigmentation-treatment/

2. https://d1wqtxts1xzle7.cloudfront.net/51351907/Clinical_
   and_instrumental_study_of_the_e20170114-2276-igefuj.
   pdf?1484410248=&response-content-disposition=inline%3B+
   filename%3DClinical_and_instrumental_study_of_the_e.
   pdf&Expires=1603955990&Signature=AFR5q6lKX85miX
   N8WOr9D3umvzkVHs2iOiKRPke3tQ16S518YqceHxwm
   0M54oOZyDHWMwrAv1MrSp4cGHktP9SDQlynrNDkq
   K7QJBMPmARgK2pHj9UijEKzy0m0LPPUELdTm4EPK
   XyM-0b0-Z4rzpAZFJVklNiEx~KaJWqEejjRVIMJgYpL13
   Vjiq~WCdqVIcbf2mvv4L-hb39M2AtDms3lymvwedVzd6v
   MaooqX6yVnW5DGwWfUJrHul0GjaQdXyoiQxJV7WWh
   AQm3S9UzM7NgjEU7FAMz7~8JYPCDRkMFZhXnQX4t
   HitiUPCABQQhudYpUwL40ENIoFxnnkNYA0A__&Key-Pair-
   Id=APKAJLOHF5GGSLRBV4ZA

3. Christos C. Zouboulis, "Acne and Sebaceous Gland Function
   Clinics in Dermatology" 22; (2004); 360–366
   http://www.klinikum-dessau.de/fileadmin/user_upload/
   Hautklinik/PDF-Files/235_clinder-acne-etiol.pdf

4. https://www.herbaldynamicsbeauty.com/blogs/herbal
   -dynamics-beauty/understanding-the-comedogenic-scale-for
   -oils-and-butters

5. https://www.ncbi.nlm.nih.gov/pmc/articles/PMC5605215/

6. https://www.hindawi.com/journals/mi/2010/858176/

7. https://www.tandfonline.com/doi/abs/10.1080/147641706
   00717704?scroll=top&needAccess=true&journalCode=ijcl20

8. https://www.ncbi.nlm.nih.gov/pmc/articles/PMC3663177/

9. http://www.isyaderm.com/dark-circles/

10. https://www.ncbi.nlm.nih.gov/pmc/articles/PMC3884927/

11. https://plasticsurgerykey.com/disturbances-of-pigmentation/

ACKNOWLEDGEMENTS

My Dad, Maninder Singh Sethi who is my hero, my Mom, Dr Nisha Kaur Sethi, who is my heart, my brothers Kavneet Singh Sethi and Teghvir Singh Sethi, who love me no matter what, my nephews, my sister-in law and my extended family who I will love forever. Thank you to my family and friends who have stood by me, and for those who were my support through rough times. Also, thank you to my mentor Dr Umesh Vohra: you taught me how to explore my field and be a good human being and a doctor.

Lastly, to all of you, my growth and perseverance is because of your support, and I carry you all in everything I do.

ABOUT THE AUTHOR

Dr Kiran Sethi, MD, is a celeb integrative skin, wellness and aesthetic physician. She has been named as one of the best skin experts in the country by *Elle, Franchise India* and other publications. Dr Sethi has written for *Vogue, Harper's Bazaar, Hindustan Times, Times of India,* and *Mint,* among others. She has also appeared on various television shows for NDTV, CNBC, India Today, Aaj Tak, to name a few. She is also a lead trainer and key opinion leader for many brands. Dr Sethi collaborates with doctors and institutions from around the world to bring a beauty from inside-out approach to her clients and followers.